Mycetoma

Dr. K. R. Joshi
M.D. (Path & Micro), Ph.D. (Path) M.N.A.M.S.
Ex. Prof. & Head, Deptt. of Microbiology
Dr. Sampurnanand Medical College, Jodhpur
Ex. Principal, Medical College, Kota

Dr. Aruna Solanki
M.D. (Path), M.D. (Micro)
Associate Professor, Deptt. of Microbiology
Dr. Sampurnanand Medical College, Jodhpur

Dr. Y. R. Joshi
M.D. (Path)
Senior Demonstrator, Deptt. of Pathology
Dr. Sampurnanand Medical College, Jodhpur

Agrobios (India)

Published by:
Agrobios (India)
Behind Nasrani Cinema
Chopasani Road, Jodhpur 342 002
Phone: 0291-642319

Published by **Agrobios (India),** Behind Nasrani Cinema, Chopasani Road, Jodhpur 342 002
Phone: 0291-642319, Email Agrobios.@vsnl.com.
Printed by H. S. Offset Printers, New Delhi.

Foreword

Mycetoma, also known as *Madurafoo*, is so named as it was first seen by Gill (1842) while working at a dispensary, at Madurai, the ancient capital of Pandyam kingdom in southern India and famous for its fantastic temples. This condition known in Ayurveda as *Pada Valmiki* existed since antiquity. The term *Mycetoma* was coined by Vandyke Carter (1860) who classified it according to the colour of the grains seen in the lesion and discharged in the pus. The term *Madurafoot* had been in the past indiscriminately used ignoring the diverse aetiologic agents and unusual sites of infection. When cultural studies yielded different causative agents, Pinoy (1913) divided Mycetoma into two types, Actinomycotic Mycetoma due to aerobic actinomycetes and Maduromycotic Mycetoma caused by true fungi. Chalmers and Archibald (1916) suggested the *Maduromycosis* for the latter. But fungi other than Madurella are known to cause Mycetoma and this condition is seen in different parts of the world, far away from Madurai. Mycetoma is not restricted to foot only or to one geographic area as suggested by the original term *Madurafoot.*

The concept of Mycetoma is thus expanded to include morphologically characteristic lesions in any part of the body, as well as the diverse aetiologic agents prevalent in different parts of the world. However, some order in classification by determining the specific causative agent and naming the lesion according to botanical terminology is now universally accepted.

This monograph summarizes the work done in India in this field. It is a comprehensive treatise on this subject, originating at the first national symposium on Mycetoma held at Jodhpur in February 1998, under the auspices of SIHAM. It covers the entire range of topics with separate chapters on each aspect of the disease, supported by references to literature. A rich collection of photographs showing the clinical conditions, tissue lesions, cultural identification of the aetiological agents and pathogenesis make this treatise useful to students and teachers of medical mycology. It is a good contribution to our knowledge in geographic pathology.

Dr. L. N. Mohapatra

Preface

A National Symposium on Mycetoma was held on 26th to 28th Feb. 1998 at the Department of Microbiology, Dr. Sampurnanand Medical College, Jodhpur. The faculty contributed in the symposium by way of deliberations and discussions. It included Microbiologists, General and Orthopedic surgeons, Pathologists and Dermatologists. At the end of the symposium, it was considered to publish the *Monograph on Mycetoma* with a view to disseminating update knowledge to the concerned. The present monograph is been published to fulfill the desire of participants and faculty members of the symposium. It covers all topics on mycetoma. As desired by most of the faculty members, special attention has been paid to incorporate a large number of clinical and microphotographs to present the varied picture of mycetoma. We have tried to update knowledge and have included two hundred and ninety four references.

The photographs included are those, which were presented during the first National Symposium on Mycetoma by various speakers, many of which are their original and others appear to be reproduced from standard books / atlas on mycology.

We feel pleasure in conveying our thanks to NAMS, DST, UGC and Principal, Dr. Sampurnanand Medical College, Jodhpur for providing financial assistance to organise the symposium and publish the monograph. We are specially thankful to Dr. L. N. Mohapatra and Dr. H.C. Gugnani for their initial financial contribution for preparing the monograph. Our special thanks to Dr. D. R. Mathur and Dr. S. S. Sankhala for providing assistance in photography.

We also wish to acknowledge our thanks to the. Agrobios (India), Jodhpur for publishing the monograph. We are also thankful to photographer Mr. Ravindra Nath for extending his co-operation in getting the cases photographed. Finally, we express our great appreciation to Mr. O. P. Solanki for his assistance during publication.

Authors

Jodhpur
January 2000

Contents

Participants

1. Dr. L. N. Mohapatra
   Ex. Dean A.I.I.M.S. New Delhi
   Director, R.M.R.C., I.C.M.R.
   Bhubaneshwar, Orissa

2. Dr. H. S. Randhawa
   Dean, Vallabh Bhai Patel Chest
   Institute, Delhi.

3. Dr. Maya Attapattu.
   Prof. & Head, Bacteriology and
   Mycology Deptt., Medical Research Institute, Sri Lanka

4. Dr. Pankaj Laxmi
   Director, Institute of Medical Microbiology, Chennai

5. Dr. K. R. Joshi
   Ex. Prof. & Head, Deptt. of Microbiology
   Ex. Principal, Medical College, Kota

6. Dr. K. K. Sharma
   Ex. Prof. & Head, Deptt. of Microbiology
   Dr. S. N. Medical College, Jodhpur
   Ex. Principal, J. L. N. Medical College, Ajmer

7. Dr. C. S. Bais
Associate Professor, Deptt of Microbiology
Medical College, Jodhpur

8. Dr. Aruna Solanki
Assistant Professor, Deptt. of Microbiology
Dr. S. N. Medical College, Jodhpur

9. Dr. P. K. Khatri
Assistant Professor, Deptt. of Microbiology
Dr. S. N. Medical College, Jodhpur

10. Dr. Sohan Singh Sankhala
Associate Professor Deptt. of Orthopaedics,
S. M. S. Medical College, Jaipur.

11. Dr. Harbans Singh
Ex. Prof. & Head. Deptt. of Surgery
Ex. Principal, Medical College, Kota

12. Dr. J. C. Sharma
Ex. Prof. & Head, Deptt. of Orthopaedics
Ex. Principal S.M.S. Medical College Jaipur.

13. Dr. Gopi Ram Agarwal
Ex. Prof. & Head, Deptt. of Radiology
Ex. Principal Medical College, Kota

14. Dr. A. M. Singhvi
Ex. Prof. & Head, Deptt. of Surgery
Dr. S.N. Medical College, Jodhpur

15. Dr. H. C. Gugnani
Prof. Vallabh Bhai Patel Chest Institute
Delhi.

16. Dr. A. Chakrabarti
Additional Professor Post Graduate
Institute of Medical Education and Research
Chandigarh

17. Dr. Gyaneshwar Kalla
Prof. & Head Deptt. of Skin and V.D.
Dr. S.N. Medical College, Jodhpur

18. Dr. D. R. Mathur
    Prof. & Head, Deptt. of Pathology
    Dr. S. N. Medical College, Jodhpur

19. Dr. M. C. R. Vyas
    Prof. & Head, Deptt. of Pathology
    Medical College, Kota

20. Dr. I. N. Ramdeo
    Ex. Prof. & Head, Deptt of Pathology
    Dr. S.N. Medical College, Jodhpur

Chapter One

History of Mycetoma

Mycetoma is a chronic progressive granulomatous exogenous infection of subcutaneous tissue characterised by swelling and presence of granules of the aetiological agent which may spread contiguously to involve adjoining skin with formation of multiple sinuses discharging pus, granules, fragments of degenerated muscles, tendons and bones.

Mycetoma is an ancient disease, mention of this disease is found in the very old Indian Vedic treatise *Atharva Veda* in which it is described as *Padvalmicum* - meaning the ant-hill of foot. Locally it is popular as *Kiri-Nagra.* According to the records of French missionaries in Pondicherry, similar disease was noticed and described as "*Fourmiliere desvers*" as early as 1714 (Ghosh and Panja 1950). The disease was described to be characterised by numerous small ulcers with communicating channels, some healing and other opening. However, as a distinct clinical entity it was first recognised by Gill in 1842 at Madurai. He described the clinical features of the disease: *characterised by marked deformity of foot with large fungal excrescenses, an offensive and ichorous discharge and involving the joints, cartilages and ligaments.* Colebrook (1846) who succeded Gill in Madurai dispensary named it as *Madura Foot.*

Wider attention was first focused on the disease by Godfrey (1846), who was first to mention the black granules of the character of coal fragments in the diseased tissue of the foot but he ignored these granules and mentioned the condition as "*Morbus tuberculosis Pedis*". Henery Van Carter (1860) a professor of Morbid Anatomy and Physiology at Grant Medical College Bombay established its fungal aetiology and coined the name Mycetoma

(*Mycos* - Fungus) implying a tumour like enlargement caused by fungal infection. In 1874, he brought out a comprehensive monograph on mycetoma "The fungus disease of India" which was in keeping with the general conviction that the disease was confined to the Indian sub-continent. He described that the foot was not the only site of infection nor was the disease localised to Madurai only. Two varieties of the disease were described - one presenting with black (*Melanoid*) granules and the other presenting with white (*Ochroid*) granules. He catalogued different colours of the grains and proposed that these represent different organisms.

Bocarro (1893) while working in Bombay made a detailed study of 100 cases of mycetoma and published his clinical and histopathological findings. In his opinion aetiological agents are presumably introduced by a minor injury. He had an opportunity to examine an inflammatory lesion round a thorn buried in tissue. In 1894 he tried to distinguished between black and white varieties of mycetoma on clinical and histopathological grounds and he thought that they were separate varieties of disease caused by different agents. He also noticed that relapsed cases resembled the original infection.

Bristowe (1871) examined grains microscopically after boiling them in liquor potassae and teasing the hyphae apart. This process also removed pigment from grains. He noted the grains consisted of hyphae and large rounded cells resembling chlamydospores. Boyce and Surveyor (1894) found that eau de javelle was better cleaning agent than liquor potassae and established that the organisms of black and white varieties were independent entities and also showed that many of the pale grains were caused by actinomycetes rather than fungi. They were also able to describe the tissue reactions associated with mycetoma i.e. hyperplasia and tissue destruction and infiltration of small round cells (probably leucocytes), macrophages and giant cells. Vincent (1894) reinforced the idea of Actinomycetes being one of the types of causal agents by isolating an organism which he named Streptothrix madurae from yellow grains in Algeria. Brumpt (1906) described a fungus isolated from black grains for which he created the new binomial Madurella mycetomi, a fungus since then proved to be the most important single cause of mycetoma. Pinoy (1913) was the first to study the actinomycotic agents. He subdivided the disease into two basic etiologic types *actinomycoses* resulting from infection with Actinomyces group and true mycetoma caused by true fungi or molds. Chalmers and Archibald (1916) and Chalmers and Christopherson (1916) modified the terminology and extended the term mycetoma to include mycotic infection producing granules in all body tissues and did not restrict it to the foot. These authors proposed the new term *maduromycosis* for what previously called as true mycetoma and sub divided the mycetoma into two groups viz (a) Actinomycotic type having grains composed of filamentous mycelia without distinct walls and without chlamydospores and (b) Maduromycosis composed of large septate mycelia with well defined walls and chlamydospores.

Gammel (1927) presented a thorough review on the subject and enumerated the species of the two classes. Mackinnon (1954, 1956) enumerated agents of actionomycotic mycetoma and maduromycosis. Descriptions of causal agents were published as they were discovered and are still being published as they are known better and better.

Until the end of 19th centaury, mycetoma was reported almost exclusively from India then the pendulum shifted to Africa for nearly three decades. Soon it was recognised that disease exists in many tropical and subtropical countries in all continents of the world between latitudes 15° South and 30° North.

In last four decades a number of reports appeared in literature regarding its prevalence in India. It has been reported from almost all states of India. A large number of cases are from west Rajasthan and Tamil Nadu.

Chapter Two

Aetiological Agents of Mycetoma

A large number of organisms have been and still being described as agents of mycetoma but attempts to keep them down to a reasonable number have been made from time to time. Carter (1860) was the first to establish the fungal etiology of mycetoma. The first attempt to classify the causative agents of mycetoma was undertaken by Chalmers and Archibald (1918), they subdivided mycetoma into two groups maduromycosis and actinomycosis. The former refer to those forms of mycetoma with grains composed of large segmented mycelial filaments possessing well defined walls, and usually also chlamydospores and the latter those forms of mycetoma with grain composed of very fine filaments. Maduromycosis is now used to describe mycetoma caused by any true fungus.

The various types of maduromycosis were differentiated according to the colour of the grains i.e. black, white or yellow and red and sub divided further on regional basis depending on the continent in which they were isolated.

Accordingly following varieties were described:

I. (a) European Black Maduromycosis

African Black Maduromycosis

Asian Black Maduromycosis

(b) European White Maduromycosis

African White Maduromycosis

Asian White Maduromycosis

(c) The Red Maduromycosis

Balfour and Archibald's Red Maduromycosis

II (a) Black Actinomycosis

(b) White or Yellow Actinomycosis

(c) Red Actinomycosis with Red (Sometimes Yellowish) grains

Gammel (1927) presented an exhaustive list of organisms reported to have caused mycetoma and added to it two new fungi which he himself isolated and named *Madurella americana* and *Madurella ikedae*. Species differentiation of the causative agents was then based on morphological differentiation. Since many of these fungi are unstable and some of these were isolated only once or some considered to be contaminants. As such in the list of causative agents were included many agents which were not causative agents and also different names were given to the same agent so Meckinnon and his associates (1954, 1956) managed to reduce many species to synonyms. Winslow and Steen (1964) proposed a balanced classification of etiological agents of mycetoma. An updated list of causative agents is given below.

I. Agents causing Eumycetoma (Maduromycetoma)

1. *Madurella mycetomatis*
2. *Madurella grisea*
3. *Exophiala jeanselmei* (*Phialophora jeanselmei*)
4. *Allescheria boydii* or *Psaudallescheria boydii* (*Petriellidium boydii*)
5. *Acremonium* species (*Cephalosporium acremonium* and *C. falciforme*)
6. *Pyrenochaeta romeroi*
7. *Leptosphaeria senegalensis* and *L. tompkinsii*.
8. *Curvularia lunata* and *C. geniculata*

9. *Neotestudina rosatii*
10. *Aspergillus nidulans*
11. *Fusarium* species

II. Agents causing Schizomycetoma

A. Agents causing Actinomycotic mycetoma

1. *Actinomadura madurae*
2. *Actinomadura pelletieri*
3. *Streptomyces somaliensis*
4. *Nocardia brasiliensis*
5. *Norcardia asteroides*
6. *Nocardia caviae*

B. Agents causing Botryomycosis

1. *Staphylococus* spp.
2. *Escherichia coli*
3. *Proteus* spp.
4. *Pseudomonas* spp.
5. *Streptococcus* spp.
6. *Actinobacillus lignieresi*

Generally, only one of the agents mentioned above cause mycetoma. Rarely more than one agents belonging to same or other groups may cause disease in same patient at different sites or at same site (Sankhala et al 1987).

The aetiological agents of mycetoma identified varies from one geographical area to other. Mathur and Agrawal (1986) from Nigeria concluded in their study that *Streptomyces somaliensis* causing mycetoma is more common in comparison to *Madurella* species. Similar were the findings of Bendle et al (1987) from Saudi Arabia. L. Opez et al (1992) from Mexico reported *Nocardia brasiliensis* 86.6% and *Actinomadura madure* 10.2%. *M. grisea* and *M. mycetomatis* recovered in least number. Castro et al (1993) studied 41 cases of mycetoma in Brazil. The cases were caused by Actinomycetes (68%) and the commonest agent was *Nocardia brasiliensis*. The true fungi were isolated in 32% cases and these were *Madurella mycetomatis, Madurella grisea* and *Scedosporium apiospermum.*

Indian studies by Desai et al (1970) from Bombay, Dasgupta and Co-workers (1974) from Pondicherry, Grueber and Kumar (1970), and Talwar and Sehgal (1979) from North India, Pankaj-laxmi and Taralaxmi (1984) from Madras had revealed predominance of actinomycotic mycetoma rather than eumycotic mycetoma whereas Koshi et al (1981) found equal incidence of both types of mycetoma from Tamil Nadu. Venugopal and Venugopal (1991) identified 73 cases of *Actinomadura madurae* from Madras. In Rajasthan, the aetiological agents of mycetoma also varies from region to region. Singhvi et al (1995) cultured aetiological agents of *Actinomycotic mycetoma* in 52% cases. Singh (1979) observed that at Bikaner out of 223 cases studied, *Madurella mycetomatis* was identified in 188 cases. Mathur et al (1979) from Jodhpur also reported higher incidence (60%) of *Madurella mycetomatis*. Similar finding were observed by Chugh et al (1975) and Joshi et al in 1987. Joshi et al (1987) studied 382 patients of mycetoma, *Madurella mycetomatis* was most common and less common agents were *Streptomyces somaliensis, Actinomadura madurae* and *Nocardia* species. The least common species were *Madurella grisea, Leptosphaeria senegalensis, Phialophora* sp., *Pseudallescheria boydii* and *Actinomadura pelletieri*. Mycetoma caused by *Nocardia* was observed significantly more in south-east region than in north-west region of Rajasthan. Sharma et al (1990) found that actinomycetes involve extrapedal sites relatively more frequently than true fungi. Chakrabarti and Singh (1998) from Chandigarh observed that out of 23 patients 56.5% were found to have actinomycotic agents while 43.5% cases were of eumycotic mycetoma with *Madurella mycetomatis* preponderance. *Madurella grisea* was found in least number, *Nocardia asteroides* and *Actinomadura madurae* were common agents of actinomycotic mycetoma.

Mycetoma caused by *Madurella grisea* has been reported in few cases from America (Mariat 1963), Brazil (Silva et al, 1991; Castro et al, 1993), Saudi Arabia (Venugopal et al, 1990), South India (Klokke 1967 and Gokhalay et al 1968) Madras (Venegopal and Venugopal 1991), Chandigarh (Chakrabarti and Singh 1998), Madura (Indira and Sirsi, 1968) and Rajasthan (Joshi et al 1971, Mathur et al 1979, Joshi et al 1987).

Actinomadura pellitieri is a rare aetiological agent of mycetoma which is also reported time to time from different regions i.e. from Africa (Verghese and Klokke 1966), Senegal, Somalia and Mexico (Mahgoub and Murray 1973), South India (Klokke et al 1968), Rajasthan (Joshi et al, 1980, 1987,

Mathur et al 1993, 1994) and Madurai (Venugopal and Venugopal 1990a and Pankajlaxmi and Taralaxmi 1990).

Nocardia species are common aetiological agents of actinomycotic mycetoma. These are *Nocardia brasiliensis, Nocardia asteroides, Nocardia caviae* and *Nocardia transvalensis*. Many workers [Rajendran and Kandhari (1989), Lopez et al (1992), Castro et al (1993), Wortman (1993), Verghese et al (1996)] isolated *Nocardia brasiliensis*. The earlier reports on mycetoma due to *N. brasiliensis* in India were by Klokke (1964) from Punjab, Sanyal and Basu (1964) and Basu et al (1974) from West Bengal, Desai et al (1970) and Mohanty et al (1982) from Maharashtra, Pankajlakshmi and Taralaksmi (1982) from South India and Rajendran and Kandhari (1988) from Delhi. *Nocardia caviae* was cultured by Dravid et al (1991) and *Nocardia asteroides* by Saraca et al (1993), Akagawa et al (1997) and Chakarbarti and Singh (1998). Mycetoma caused by *Nocardia transvalensis* has been reported by Mishra et al (1980), Gugnani et al (1983) and Mirza and Campbell (1994). Sharma et al (1987) reported mycetoma caused by *Streptomyces somaliensis*.

Other rarely reported eumycotic agents are *Aspergillus nidulans* (Baylet et al 1968, Mahgoub 1971, Joshi et al 1985). *Aspergillus flavus* (Witzig et al 1996), *Exophiala jeanselmei* (Talwar and Sehgal, 1979; Thammayya and Sanyal 1980; Hemashettar et al 1986; Neurmeister et al 1995), *Phialophora cyanescens* (de Hoog et al 1993), *Phialophora verrucosa* (Turiansky et al 1995), *Cladosporium normodendrum* (Buiting et al 1993), *Acremonium* (Fincher et al 1991), *Leptosphaeria tompkinsii* (Venugopal and Venugopal 1990b), *Cylindrocarpon destructans* (Zoutman and Sigler 1991), *Scedosporium apiospermum* (Castro et al 1993). *Pseudallescheria boydii* (Venugopal and Venugopal 1995). *Arthrographis kalarae* (Degavri et al 1997), *Curvularia lunata* (Elad et al 1991), Fusarium (Baudraz - Rossel et al 1992, Buiting et al 1993).

Pulmonary mycetoma caused by *Candida albicans* is also reported for the first time by Shelly et al (1996) and pulmonary mycetoma like lesion produced by *C. tropicalis* has also been reported by Prats et al (1995).

Botryomycosis is a rare and chronic but treatable form of mycetoma. It is caused by persistent bacterial infection and is distinguished by formation of grain and multiple sinuses in the skin. The name granular bacteriosis has also been proposed for this disease. Clinically and histologically it resembles mycetoma and actinomycosis. The bacteria like *Staphylococci, Escherichia coli, Proteus* species, *Pseudomonas aeruginosa*, non haemolytic *Streptococci, Actinobacillus ligneiresi, Bacteroides* and *Rhodococcus* species are responsible for botrymycosis (Chander 1995). It is most usually caused by *Staphylococcus aureus* (Findlay and Vismer 1990, Ellerbe et. al 1997) Microscopically the organisms appear to be encapsulated in granules, which are thought to protect them from the effects of standard courses of antibiotics.

The lesions may develop any where on the skin, head, pinnae, hands and feet. The disseminated form may occur. Several cases have been reported in children with cystic fibrosis, following surgery, skin abrasions, lacerations and piercing of ear in debilitated patients (Chander 1996).

Chapter Three

Epidemiology of Mycetoma

GEOGRAPHICAL DISTRIBUTION

Mycetoma has been reported from almost all over the world., The disease predominantly occurs in tropical and subtropical countries and few cases were reported from temperate region. A hazy picture of epidemiology of mycetoma in different parts of the world is available mainly from the reported incidence of mycetoma by various workers notably Abbot (1954, 1956) Lynch (1964) and Murray (1960) from Sudan; Green and Adams in 1964 from United States, Latapi and Ortize (1963) from Mexico, Garden et al (1966) from Columbia, Flavial (1958) from Argentina, Chadfield (1964), Murray and Holt (1964) and Baxter et al (1966) from United Kingdom, Reifferschied and Seeliger (1955) from Germany, Cooray (1962) and Nityananda (1962) from Ceylon; Reyes (1963) from Philippines, Fukushire and Mariat (1965) and Akagawa et al (1997) from Japan, Brounst et al (1962) from Lebanon, Oyston (1961) from Thailand, Baylet et al (1961) from Senegal and West Africa, Orio et al (1963), Mahgoub and Murray (1973) and Destombes et al (1977) from Somalia and Segretain and Destombes (1963) from North America, El mofti et al (1965) from Egypt, Wilson (1965) from Uganda, Mathur and Agarwal (1986) from Nigeria, Bendle et al (1987) from Saudi Arabia, Huerre et al (1991) from New Caledonia, Wanke et al (1992) and Castro et al el (1993) from Brazil, L. Opez Mart et al (1992) and Southern (1996) from Mexico, Yu et al (1993) from Yemen, Mirza and Campbell (1994) from Pakistan, Turiansky et al (1995) from Washington D.C. and Sakand et al (1998) from Burkina Faso.

Mariat attempted to make world wise survey of mycetoma in 1963. He published his data originally consisting of 854 cases collected from 77 replies from questionnaire to 131 workers in different areas of world between 1940 and 1960. In his data Sudan and India were not included as no returns were made from these countries. Desai et al in (1970) from Bombay modified report of Mariat (1963) with addition of reports which they could gathered from other areas and reported 5322 cases including India, Africa and Madagasear.

A survey was carried out in Mexico by L Opez Mart et al in 1992 to determine the incidence and epidemiology of mycetoma. Data was collected from a total of 2105 cases of mycetoma throughout 30 years period (1956-1985) with an average incidence of 70 cases per year. The geographical distribution with in Mexico revealed that the states with the highest incidence were Jalisco, Nuevo Leon, San luis Potosi, Morelos and Guerrero. Castro et al (1993) done retrospective study of 41 cases seen in Brazil. Most of the patients came from rural areas in North Eastern region of the country and worked as field labourers. Yu et al (1993) studied mycetoma in Northen Yemen and found that it has same endemic area for mycetoma as estern Africa.

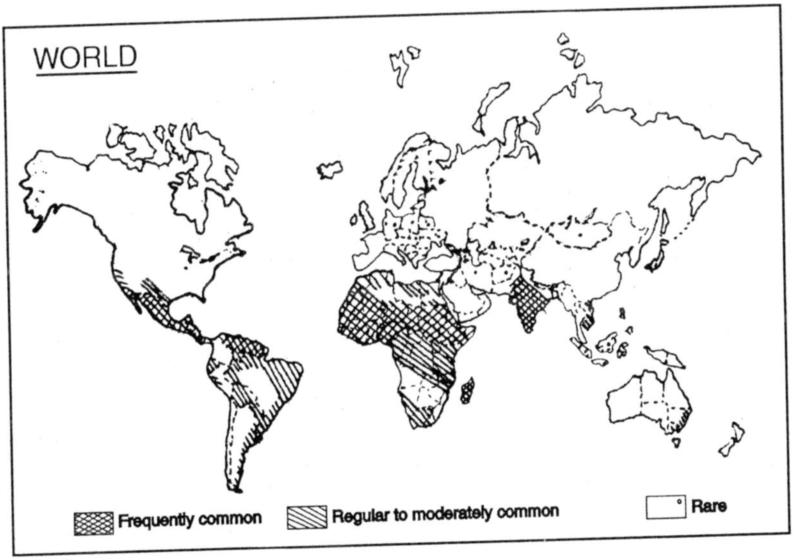

Fig. 1: Endemic area of mycetoma in world.

Mycetoma predominantly occurs in a band between lattitudes of 10° and 28°N which includes Mexico, Central and South-America, Venezuela. Senegal, Aregntina, Chand, Nigeria, Sudan, Saudi Arabia and India. Cases are being reported from time to time outside this zone.

Mycetoma in India

The disease is prevalent in almost all parts of India as reported originally by Carter (1860). The publications from various parts of India include Bengal (Ghosh et al 1950, Kakoti and Dey 1956, Panja and Choudhary 1958, Benerjee et al 1961, Sanyal and Basu 1964), Maharastra and Gujrat (Mankodi and Kanvindo 1970, Desai et al 1970, Bapat and Pandit 1991), Tamil Nadu and Andra Pradesh (Murti and Padmavati 1963, Verghese and Klokke 1966, Klokke et al 1968), Punjab and Delhi (Klokke 1964, Mahapatra and Bhargava 1967), Haryana (Chugh 1975), Poona (Tambaku and Sengupta 1969), Jabalpur (Chouhan and Agarwal 1969), Vishakapatanam (Reddy et al 1972), Pondicherry (Dasgupta et al 1974). Guntoor (Murli and Padmavati, 1963), Madras (Pankajlaxmi and Taralaxmi 1984, Venugopal et al 1977, 1990, 1991, 1993), Chandigarh (Talwar and Sehgal 1979, Chakarbarti and Singh 1998) and Rajasthan (Andleigh 1954, Joshi 1973, 1980, 1985, 1987; Singh 1979; Sharma 1987, 1988, 1990; Mathur 1979, 1993, 1994; Singhvi 1995).

Vanbreuseghen (1967) stated that mycetoma occurs in places where rainfall is 50-500 mm with temperature ranging from 15°-25°C but in India conditions are different where distribution of mycetoma is recorded in widely variable geographic conditions. In India actinomycotic mycetoma is more common in South India and North India (Desai et al 1970, Klokke et al 1968, Pankajlaxmi and Taralaxmi 1984, Talwar and Sehgal 1979, Chakrabarti and Singh 1998), whereas eumycetoma is more common in North-West part of India i.e. Rajasthan (Singh 1979, Joshi et al 1987). Maximum cases of mycetoma has been reported from Rajasthan and Tamil Nadu.

Actually a variety of environmental and social factors, such as rainfall, temperature, soil, abundance of thorny sharp vegetable material on land capable of inoculation of mycetoma agents and habit of walking barefoot, all combine to produce a favourable milieu for this disease.

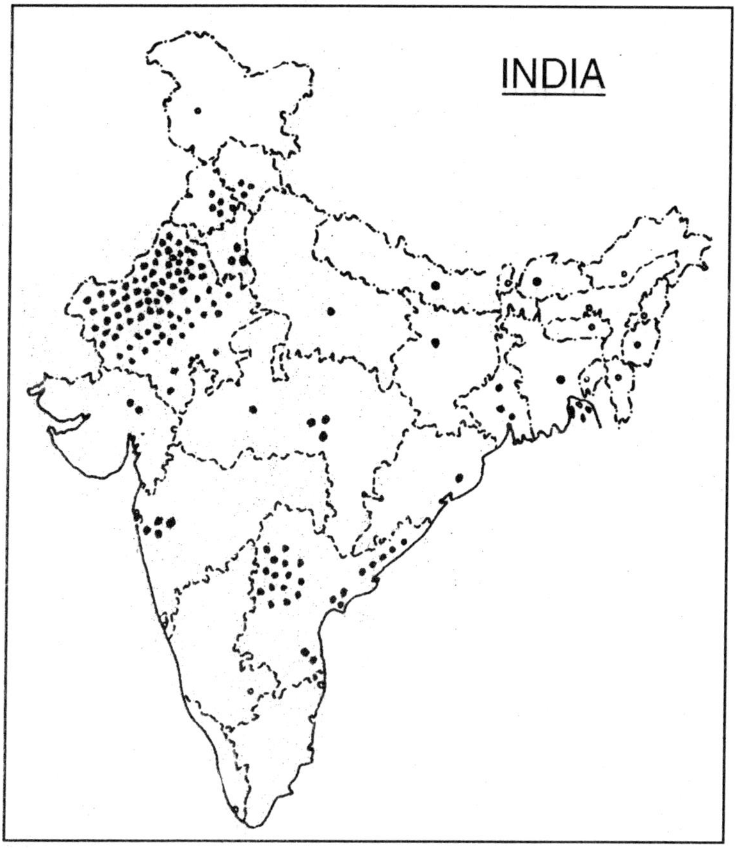

Fig. 2: Prevalence of mycetoma in India

Mycetoma in Rajasthan

Mycetoma is endemic in Rajasthan. The mycetoma cases reported from this region include studies of Andleigh (1954), Sran et al (1972), Singh (1976, 1979), Joshi et al (1973, 1980, 1985, 1987), Sharma et al (1987, 1988 and 1990), Mathur et al (1979, 1993, 1994), Singhvi et al (1995). Singh (1979) reported 262 cases of mycetoma. According to his study 20-25 cases of mycetoma were added to A.G. Hospitals of S.P. Medical College, Bikaner every year. Mathur et al (1979) reported a series of 133 patients of mycetoma treated at A.G. Group of Hospital, S.N. Medical College, Jodhpur from 1968 to 1978. Joshi et al (1987) did histological identification of mycetoma in 382 patients studied who attended the hospital attached to five medical colleges in Rajasthan at Jaipur, Ajmer, Bikaner and Jodhpur and Udaipur. Based upon the nature of soil and rainfall the state has been divided into three arbitrary regions (i) North-west desert region consisting of districts Ganganagar, Bikaner, Churu, Jaisalmer, Barmer and Jodhpur with annual rainfall of less than 350mm; (ii) Central region of plains consisting of districts Jhunjhunu, Sikar, Jaipur, Nagour, Ajmer, Pali, Jalore wtih rainfal of 350-550mm; (iii) South-East Arawali Hill region consisting of Sawai-Madhopur, Bhilwara, Chittorgarh, Udaipur, Sirohi, Dungarpur and Bhanswara with rainfall more than 600mm. The disease was most prevalent in north-west region which accounted for two third of patients. The ratio of eumycetoma to actinomycotic mycetoma was 3.2:1, 1.5:1 and 1:2 in north-west, central and south-east regions of state respectively. Mycetoma caused by Nocardia species was observed to be significantly more in south-east region and least in north-west region. Eumycetoma accounted for 71% of mycetoma in their study which correlates with earlier observations at Bikaner (Singh 1979) and Jodhpur (Mathur et al 1979). However, higher prevalence of actinomycotic mycetoma was observed by Singhvi et al (1995) at Jodhpur from extrapedal site. According to Joshi et al (1987) differences in prevalence of the causative agents may be related to the annual rainfall / or to the nature of soil in these regions.

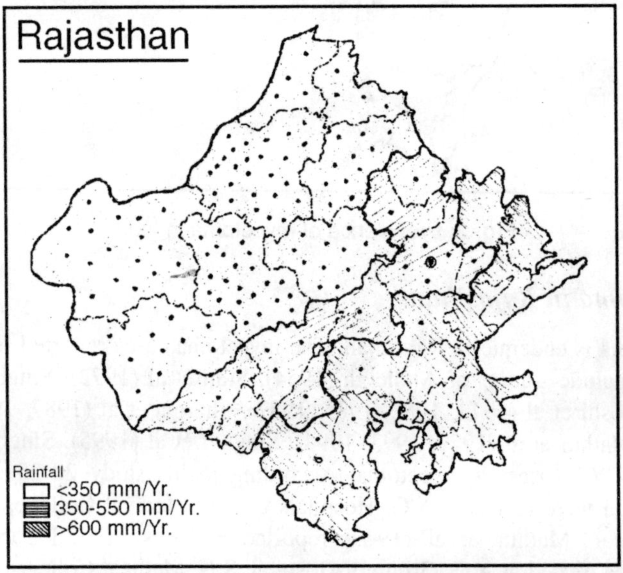

Fig. 3: Distribution of cases of mycetoma in Rajasthan

AGE, SEX AND OCCUPATIONAL INCIDENCE IN MYCETOMA

Age

The disease occurs most frequently between the ages 20 and 40 years (Bocorro 1893, Gonzalez Ochoa, 1962, DasGupta et al 1973, Venugopal et al 1977, Singh 1979, Mathur et al 1979, Sharma et al 1988, Philippon et al 1992, L. Opez et al 1992, Fahal and Hassan 1992, Castro et al 1993, Singhvi et al 1995 and Chakarbarti and Singh 1998). Bendle et al (1987) reported cases from 18 to 74 years with average age 42 year. The importance of age group 20-40 years can be explained by the fact that during this period of life the person is highly active and works hard thereby exposing himself and becoming more vulnerable to thorn prick or trauma and injury.

Sex

Mycetoma is seen more frequently in men than women. The male and female ratio observed by Abbott (1956) and Lynch (1964) in Sudan was 5:1, whereas the ratio given by Green and Adams (1964) in United States was 3.5:1. Bendle et al (1987) in Saudi Arabia observed this ratio 9:1. L. Opez et al (1992) found 76.1% male and 23.9% female mycetoma patients while studying 2105 cases in Mexico.

The sex ratio of male to female patients observed by workers in India are 4:1 by Bocarro (1893) and Banerjee et al (1961), 2:1 by Chauhan and Agarwal (1969), 3:1 by Das Gupta et al (1974), 6:1 by Sran et al (1973), 7:1 by Chugh et al (1975), 5:1 by Venugopal et al (1977), 4:1 by Singh (1979), 3:1 by Mathur et al (1979), 2:1 by Sharma et al (1988) and Pankajlaxmi and Taralaxmi (1984) and nearly 1:1 by Chakarbarti and Singh (1998). Maiti and Halder (1998) observed that there is significant difference in male female ratio regarding exposed and covered parts of body. The "covered area" cases had almost equal incidence of mycetoma in both sexes. But in "exposed area", preponderance of male cases were seen. The higher incidence of mycetoma in men may be due to a more frequent risk of exposure related to their field work. This at least seems to be unlikely in India where females works equally hard in fields and as labourer. It is likely that females have some sort of protective mechanism against the entry and / or proliferation of causative organisms in their body. Though there is no such single study of last three decades from same region. The point worth noting from available studies is that the male-female ratio is diminishing.

Occupation

Occupational incidence reveals that disease occurs more commonly in farmers, field labourers or herdmen who come in contact with the soil in endemic areas where fungal spores causing mycetoma are prevalent. Similar observation was made by Abbott (1956) and Lynch (1964), Desai et al (1970), Sran et al (1973), Singh (1979) and Sharma et al (1988). L. Opez et al (1992) found disease in females who are housewives with rural residence. Sran et al (1973) observed that the suffered females were house wives of farmers. Castro et al (1993) also observed disease common in land workers, who are frequently exposed to minor penetrating trauma. In endemic areas disease is also seen in people from other occupations e.g. drivers, carpenters or builders. However, the disease has been reported in all works of life.

SITE OF PREDILECTION IN MYCETOMA

The analysis of literature revealed that the foot to be commonest site of mycetoma, recalling the early name, Madura foot (Abbott 1956, Lynch, 1964, Desai et al 1970, Mahgoub and Murray 1973, Sran et al 1973, Singh 1979, Mathur et al 1979, Pankajlaxmi and Taralaxmi 1984, L. Opez et al 1992, Chakarbarti and Singh 1998, Maiti and Halder 1998). Mycetoma of foot appears more particularly on the dorsum of forefoot, toe webs and sole.

Various studies indicate that extra pedal mycetoma is not uncommon and its incidence varies from 10 to 40%. Extra pedal mycetoma usually affect those parts of body that comes in contact with soil while working in the field like hands, buttocks, back, perineum etc. Mycetoma of scalp is due to habit of carrying field goods on head. Some of the sites of extra pedal mycetoma reported in literature includes eyelid (Aldridge and Krik 1940), Testicle (Clarke 1953), Vulva (Medawi Cited by Lynch 1964), Lymphnode (Oyston 1961 and Hassan and Mahgoub 1972), Buttocks and Perineum (Chhabra and Chugh 1976, Singh 1976, Mathur et al 1979, Singhvi et al 1995, Maiti and Halder 1998), Upper extrimities (Sran and Joshi 1972, Desai et al 1970, Singh 1979, Mathur 1979, Sharma et al 1988, Siano et al 1990, L. Opez et al 1992, Singhvi et al 1995, Anandi et al 1997, Maiti and Halder 1998), Middle ear cleft (Chhangani et al 1972), Jaw (Singhvi et al 1995), Scalp (Frey 1976, Singh 1979, Pankajlaxmi and Taralaxmi, 1990 Singhvi et al 1995). Trunk (L.Opez et al 1992, Gupta et al 1990 and Chakrabarti and Singh 1998), Vertebral column (Zaias 1969), Lung (Uppal et al 1993) and Neck (Singhvi et al 1995, Maiti and Halder 1998).

SOURCE AND MODE OF INFECTION IN MYCETOMA

Mycetoma is not a contagious disease and the source of infection is exogenous. It is generally believed that the introduction of organisms to the body has probably traumatic basis. The infection occurs by accidental, traumatic subcutaneous implantation of aetiological agents from its saprobic source by thorns or splinters or nails. It is a common feature that mycetoma is endemic in areas where the vegetation comprises principally of thorny trees and persons walk or work in field bare footed and farmers work with hands without protection. The role of thorn prick in the causation of mycetoma has been emphasised by many workers (Bocarro 1893, Gammel 1927, Abbott 1956, Lynch 1964, Singh 1976, 1979, Mathur et al 1979, Mathur and Agarwal 1986, Singhvi et al 1995). In a few cases thorn embedded in mycetoma have also been recorded.

Other than thorn prick, minor abrasions and trauma to skin also play important role in introduction of aetiological agents into subcutaneous tissue. History of trauma prior to disease has been reported by many workers (Lynch 1964, Singh 1976, 1979, Mathur and Agarwal 1986, Joshi et al 1985, Siano et al 1990, Wanke et al 1992, Singhvi et al 1995).

Singh (1976,79) postulated that mycetoma of perineum is probably due to working of farmers in squatting position and wearing inadequate cloths around groin thereby subjected to injuries by thorns and splinters. Cleaning of anal region after defecation with sand, a common practice in villagers, is another factor which causes minor abrasions allowing entry of aetiological agents of mycetoma.

Use of wicks (pieces of straw from field soil) for removal of wax from ear is a common feature among rural folk this may be responsible for entry of agents leading to mycetoma of middle ear (Chhangani et al 1972, Singh et al 1979). Similarly mycetoma of back is due to habit of carrying goods like wood, bags of grains, stones or other articles contaminated with soil on aforesaid areas which produces minor abrasions through which organisms gain entry (Singh et al 1979 and Joshi et al 1985). History of guinea worm extraction has been noticed by few workers (Singh 1979 and Singhvi et al 1995) prior to development of mycetoma.

Several studies have been done to isolate the causative organism of mycetoma from thorns, vegetations and soil. Abbott (1954) found that mycetoma granules can survive in soil and *M. mycetomatis* is able to grow on soil extract agar. The first mycetoma causing organism to be isolated from soil was *Nocardia asteroides*. *Nocardia* species causing mycetoma has been isolated from soil by various workers from Philippines (Reyes 1963), from Delhi (Kumar and Mohapatra 1968), from Haryana (Malik et al 1982) and from Punjab (Singh and Sandhu 1985).

Singhvi et al (1995a) studied prevalence of mycetoma causing fungi in soil and thorns in Jodhpur region. Recovery rate of fungi from soil was 25.24%. *Nocardia*, *Madurella* and *Fusarium* were isolated in the maximum number and Streptomyces in least number of samples.

The relation between thorn and mycetoma has been noted by several workers (Bocarro 1909, Gammel 1927, Abbott 1954, Rey 1961). The agents of mycetoma may live saprophytically on thorns which actually introduce the infecting agent when they penetrates. It is also likely that agents infect thorns and the infected thorn remain implanted in subcutaneous tissue to initiate foreign body granuloma and subsequently the agents invade the host tissue to produce the lesion. It is a fact that where mycetoma is endemic thorny trees are plentiful and quite often surgeons and pathologists have found thorns embedded in mycetoma lesions. Segretain and Mariat (1969) have isolated *Leptosphaeria senegalensis* in abundance from thorns in Senegal. Singhvi et al (1995a) isolated fungus causing mycetoma in 16.06% of thorns cultured. *Madurella* and *Fusarium* were the commonest isolates and Nocardia, *Pseudallescheria boydii* and Philophora were also isolated in some samples. Isolation rate varied from different types of thorns. Prosopis juliphora (English babul), *Acacia nylotica* (Desi babul), *Ziziphus numularia* (Bair) and *Prosopis cineraria* (Khejdi) thorns are rich in these pathogenic fungi.

Chapter Four

Clinical Presentation of Mycetoma

The clinical picture of mycetoma, despite of its diverse aetiological agents, falls with in a single general clinical type with many common features in most of the cases but may differ in individual cases, depending upon aetiological agents, duration and site of the primary development. Mycetoma is relatively painless, locally invasive, indolent tumor like lesion. The hall marks of mycetoma are :

a) Tumor and tumefication

b) Draining sinuses

c) Presence of micro-colonies of the causal organism termed 'grains' in the discharge or tissue.

Tumor

Mycetoma usually starts as a small firm, painless subcutaneous nodule. In maduromycetoma, the lesion progresses slowly, the swelling remains fairly localized. The tumor grows both towards the skin and inwards into the tissue. The surrounding anatomical arrangement of various structures is not disturbed till late in the course of the disease. In actinomycotic mycetoma the tumor mass has an ill defined margins and tends to merge into the surrounding tissue (Mahgoub and Murray 1973). Sometimes the lesion is well defined and capsulated. What helps to form capsule around the lesion is not known. It may be due to local host factors or by production of some specific enzymes or substances by the particular strain of causative organism or as a result of immunological response.

Sinuses

Sinus formation is preceded by a small bleb or blister which rupture and discharge serosanguinous fluid with grains. Old sinuses heal and close up but new open at other site. In actinomycotoic mycetoma, sinuses appear early and there is superadded bacterial infection resulting in pus formation and a serosanguinous discharge (Mahgoub and Murray 1973)

Grains

The discharge of grains or granules from sinuses is diagnostic of mycetoma, their colour, size, shape and consistency are of considerable value for the diagnosis of the species. The colour of grains in mycetoma is usually as -

White to yellow	*Cephalosporium, Pseudallescheria boydii, Neotestudina rosatii, Fusarium moniliformis, Actinomadura madurae, Streptomyces somaliensis, Nocardia* species and grains of botryomycosis.
Brown to black	*Madurella mycetomatis, M. grisea, Exophiala jeanselmei, Pyrenochaeta romeroi, Leptosphaeria senegalensis,* and *Curvularia geniculata.*
Red to Pink	*Actinomadura pelletieri.*

In mycetoma of foot, the skin looses its normal texture, it becomes thickened, pigmented and get fixed to subcutaneous tissue. The swelling is non-pitting and painless. But in 10-18% of cases pain may be due to secondary bacterial infection or to bone involvement. The lesion results in a characteristic convex sole and foot becomes broad. Even if the sinuses are absent the classical appearance of the foot may be suggestive of mycetoma.

The lesions of mycetoma present two different types of clinical appearance, one that these are invasive, infiltrative and have diffuse involvement and others may have more of superficial spread. It is difficult to explain what makes mycetoma to invade deeper tissue. It may be due to some sort of enzymatic action.

Constitutional symptoms are uncommon but whenever they are observed, are as a result of bacterial infection of open sinuses. No constitutional symptoms are seen in encapsulated lesion. Lymphoedema and varicose veins are rarely observed in infected patients (Fahal and Hassan 1992). Some of the patients with advanced mycetoma may show cachexia and secondary anaemia but this is often due to malnutrition engendered by a reduced capacity to work effectively.

The deformities and disability in advanced cases of prolonged duration are not uncommon. Mycetoma particularly eumycetoma at unusual places such as middle ear, perianal or neck regions are fatal.

Perianal involvement by mycetoma is not uncommon in Rajasthan. Attention to fistula in ano caused by mycetoma was first focused by Singh (1976). This adds a new cause to aetiology of fistula in ano. Thus unware clinician may easily miss the diagnosis. Recurrence in this region is extremely common as complete excision is practically impossible. Moreover, most of the reported lesions were caused by *M. mycetomatis* which responds poorly to medical treatment. Lesions in this region may vary from localized to very extensive involvement.

Mycetoma in general do not respect anatomical barriers. However, mycetoma of hand presents a different clinical picture resembling pyogenic infections of hand and remains confined to anatomical compartments till late. There may be localization of mycetoma lesions to phalanges, interdigital space, palm and synovial sheath. In later stages it produces a painful crippled and deformed hand when it extensively involves the soft tissues and bones of hand and even destroys the joints.

The variation from usual clinical presentation is not uncommon (Singh 1979) which may be related to an etiological agent, age of lesion, anatomical location, local or host factors, previous medical care and to the shape, size and colour of granules. These unusual lesions includes encapsulated, very well defined tumors, mass resembling a benign tumor or cyst or chronic abscess etc. These lesions are most often without sinuses and pose a diagnostic problem. The diagnosis of such atypical cases may be suspected if they meet the following criteria (Singh 1979):

i) Patients belongs to endemic area.

ii) Duration of swelling is of years.

iii) A fairly well defined painless swelling with variable consistency.

iv) Patient often belong to blood group 'O'.

v) Demonstration of granules in aspirate or biopsy confirms the diagnosis.

Clinical Staging of Mycetoma

Classical clinical presentation of tumor mass with sinuses, discharging granules is an usual finding in most of the cases of mycetoma. Few cases are presented with atypical features, in them diagnosis is difficult on clinical grounds. These cases can only be diagnosed by examining the sections of specimen grossly and histopathologically or in some cases by culture. A method of clinical staging was evolved by Singh (1998). According to him it has worked well in studying the natural behaviour and progress of the disease, planning treatment, predicting prognosis and rendering advise to patients.

The method of clinical staging was evolved on account of its similarity of this disease to clinical behaviour of cancer in certain aspects e.g.:

1. Aggressive biological behaviour.
2. No tissue respect as its lesions invade all structures.
3. Hardly any pain till late.
4. Lymphatic spread (though rare).
5. Blood borne metastasis (possibly).
6. Poor protective immunological response.
7. Surgery is the main treatment due to lack of established chemotherapy.
8. Recurrence is very common and sometimes even after radical surgery (amputation).
9. Cure is elusive.
10. Significant morbidity and mortality.

On account of so many similarities to cancer it was thought that T.N.M. classification could be applied with some modifications. In T.N.M. classification, T- represents the size of tumor, but in mycetoma, T is considered to represent the depth of invasion of the mass rather than its size, N- stands for regional lymph node involvement and M for distance metastasis.

Extent of Invasion of Tumor Like Mass (T)

T is subdivided into further subgroups similar to TNM classification used for cancer cases i.e. T1a localized encapsulated cystic masses categorised under this heading cases are rarely reported. These cases had uncommon type of lesions restricted to subcutaneous tissue.

- T1b- localized diffuse soft tissue lesion involving superficial to deep fascial plane with well defined margins.
- T1 lesions accounted for 6.4% of all cases of mycetoma, studied by Singh (1998). These lesions can be easily excised. T1a lesions do not invade or spread for long. Singh (1998) recorded such lesion of 16 years duration without ill effects, However, trauma may rupture capsule and allow invasion. T1b lesions also remain localized for long however, invasion occurs eventually.
- T2 allows invasion: These mycetoma could only be recognised at the time of incision and drainage. These are also subdivided into two
- T2a - Chronic abscess type of lesion with extension to muscle.
- T2b - localized soft tissue lesion with ill defined margin and extension to muscles.
- T2 lesions should be widely excised under tourniquet to prevent recurrences. Singh (1998) found 25.5% of T2 lesions of all cases of mycetoma studied.
- T3 accounts for large number of cases (59.7%). These lesions are further sub divided into T3a, T3b, and T3c.
- T3a - These are infiltrative lesions. Extension of soft tissue mycetomas in between the bones without their involvement such as in hand or foot are example of such lesions. Clinically lesions are fixed to deeper structures but x-ray of the part shows normal bones.
- T3b - Bone involvement is secondary to soft tissue.
- T3c - Primary bone or joint involvement is present. T3 mycetomas are also curable but demands radical surgery.
- T4 - These are most aggressive lesions and often lead to death in a short time. The examples of these lesions are mycetomas of scalp, paranasal sinuses, middle ear, mycetoma at back involving spines, mycetoma of chest and perineum. Emmon et al (1977) also stated that mycetoma of scalp are invariably fatal.

- T4 lesions are extensive and invasive lesions of soft tissues or bones or both and there is often distant metastasis to lymph nodes, bone and viscera. Such lesions are not common (10.90%).

The status of lymph node involvement, distant metastasis and recurrence of mycetoma also assigned similar status to cancer. It is true that blood and lymph node involvement was not frequent in mycetoma and blood borne metastasis were uncommon but they do occur, thereby putting mycetoma at par with cancer of low magnitute.

Lymph node involvement (N)

Lymph node involvement (N) is further divided into N0, N1, N2 and N3.

N0 - No lymph node involvement is seen.

N1 - Regional lymph nodes involved but nodes are mobile.

N2 - Regional lymph nodes involvement but nodes are fixed.

N3 - Other than regional lymph nodes involvement is seen.

Out of 310 cases of mycetoma, Singh (1998) noted regional lymph nodes metastasis only in 7 cases. Lymph node involvement other than regional lymph node was not seen.

Distant metastasis (M)

It was recorded as M0 - No distant metastasis and M1 - Distant metastasis to bone and visera.

Only in one case distant metastasis was noted and recurrence was noted in 15.48% of cases.

Chapter Five

Pathogenesis of Mycetoma

There are number of evidences to connect mycetoma with implantation of micro-organisms from the environment coupled with series of adaptive mechanisms which are beneficial for the survival of organism in human body.

Bidie (1862) believed that grains from mycetoma cases are produced by fungi that had entered in the body as spores. Bocarro (1893) found a thorn embedded in inflammatory mass of the lesion of mycetoma and he proposed that causative agent was usually introduced by minor injury. Some of the causative fungi have been isolated from the natural environment e.g. *Leptosphaeria senegalensis* has been identified in the natural environment in *Acacia* thorn (Segretain and Mariat, 1969). It is some times possible to see plant material probably originating from a thorn in some lesion of mycetoma (Cameron et al 1973). Basset and co-workers (1965) removed thorn material from two cases and cultured *L. senegalensis* from one and *Pyrenochaeta romeroi* from the other.

There is no evidence to suggest that infection is specifically associated with a host immune status, although some patients have defective T-lymphocyte mediated responses to fungi, these have been described in those with extensive disease, suggesting that these may have followed rather caused the infection (Mahgoub et al 1978). Other investigators have failed to find any changes in T-lymphocyte function in patients with disease (Bendle et al 1987). There is also no change in immune function or association with immune deficiency however, one study revealed high frequency of diabetes mellitus amongst patients of mycetoma (Hay and MacKenzie 1983). This has not been mentioned by others (Mahgoub and Murray 1973). On the other hand there are evidences that fungi may develop a number of different adaptive changes in vivo, such as cell wall reduplication or unfolding of cytoskeleton or deposition of extra or intracellular melanin all of which may adversely affect the ability of the host inflammatory response to destroy the organism. Electron microscopy of grains of eumycetoma revealed cell wall reduplication giving rise to an onion-skin appearance around cells (Hay and Collins 1983, Wethered et al 1987). This appears to follow intrahyphal growth of mycelial elements. Adjacent cell wall also fuse, particularly at rim of grain where there is also deposition of human immunoglobin. In case of *M. mycetomatis*, cells within grain may be surrounded by electron-dense homogenous material and fungal melanin. This is very resistant to physical extremes and is difficult to section using microtome (Findlay and Vismer 1987). It is thought to provide a protection for living cell within the fungal grain. It has been demonstrated that *Streptomyces somaliensis* produces an extracellular protease that affects the ability of macrophages in vitro to kill bacteria (Nasher et al 1987). So far there is very little evidences regarding immunomodulation caused by fungi of mycetoma (Leslie et al 1998).

Chapter Six

Modes of Spread of Mycetoma

Mycetoma is exogenous in origin. Once aetiological agent is implanted, lesion continue to grow, irrespective of the type of organism. The modes of spread may be:

1. Locally: The mycetoma lesion spreads in all directions and destroys whatever comes in its way. This spread is by continuity and contiguity but tendons and nerves are usually not affected. This is most usual mode of spread. The various views have been expressed stating that it spreads along fascial planes by the pressure and movements of muscles (Lynch, 1964). The spread can be through giant cells and macrophages which may ingest the causative organism and wander in tissue where they die and may liberate the organism. This seems justifiable as giant cells containing causative organism may be demonstrated in histological sections. The spread can be due to associated suppuration (Fahal and Hassan, 1992).

2. Lymphatic spread has received considerable attention by Abbott (1956), Hassan and Mahgoub (1972), Mahgoub and Murray (1973), Singh (1973) and Bendle et al (1987). This type of spread is more common in actinomycetoma. The possibilities of spread along lymphatics are many folds. The causative organism may enter the medium or large size lymphatics or lymphatics may dilate as a result of mycetoma and then organism gain entry through them. Another possibility is that the causative organisms reach nodes by permeation. But to date neither the organism, nor the grains have been demonstrated in lymphatics. Moreover, the size of granules is much larger than the lymphatics.

The regional nodes are genuinely involved in 1 to 3% of cases (Fahal and Hassan 1992). The other causes of regional lymphnode enlargement are secondary infection or immunological response.

3. The blood spread to date has not been documented as repeated blood culture do not show any evidence of causative organism of mycetoma (Singh, 1998). However, the theory of haematogenous spread proposed by Kulowaski and Stovall (1947) and Abbott (1956) can explain deep seated visceral or primary bone lesions. Cases of dissemination of infection due to *Nocardia brasiliensis* have been reported by Diamont and Bennet (1973) and Krassik et al (1976).

4. Spread along the bone marrow is not defined in the literature. But this mode of spread cannot be denied. When amputation below knee is done for mycetoma of ankle region the recurrence of stump is not uncommon. However, doubt exists that this recurrence may be through soft tissue, lymphatics or bone.

Chapter Seven

Radiology of Mycetoma

The radiological findings in mycetoma are sufficiently characteristic either to permit confirmation of a clinical diagnosis or when clinical picture is atypical it helps in locating the mycetoma lesion. Apart from identifying bone lesions, it is of great value in differentiation of type and different aetiological agents of mycetoma which indicate the line of treatment.

The most useful examination which provides information about bone invasion is plain radiography (Lewall et al 1985). Presence or absence of bone involvement depends upon the duration of illness. Joshi et al (1980) found no bone invasion in a mycetoma case as it was seen in early stage of disease before any bone invasion could occur.

Davis (1958) and Crockett (1968) had good description as -

1. Deeper soft tissue swelling could be nodular or diffuse in nature.
2. Second (Distal) row of tarsals or bases of adjoining metatarsals were the commonest sites of earlier bone involvement. Even head and shaft of metatarsals could be involved with phalanges. Amorphus bone expansion was seen in skull bones. There was diffuse thickening with loss of detailed bone structures associated with general increase in bone density.
3. Earlier bone changes were loss of definition in the cortical margins (usually the articular margins) of affected bone followed later by ragged erosion of cortex from without (but occasionally smooth) and formation of crypts representing the mouths of the sinuses.

4. Endosteal bone cavitation was seen where cystic cavities were present. These cavities were small and numerous in actinomycetomas and large and few in maduromycetoma.

5. Periosteal reaction in the form of spicules of bone upto 1cm in length projecting perpendicular to the line of cortex. It looks like uneven bristles of a partly worn brush (ragged palisade) and even "Sunray appearance" rarely linear or "Onion peel appearance" may be seen.

6. Spongiosa showed amorphus sclerosis with loss of normal trabecular pattern. Within the sclerosed spongiosa and sometimes extending through the cortex, multiple sinuses are often seen as small rounded or irregular translucent areas of 3-10mm size.

7. Dense spongiosa with its translucent areas and irregular eating away in advanced cases appeared as a "blob of melting snow".

8. Regional distal osteoporosis was observed which may be due to interference with blood supply as a result of pressure.

9. As disease progress, the bones shrinks in size, the gap between two adjacent bone increases eg. widening of intermetatarsal spaces.

10. Typical sequstra were absent but occasionally wisps of bone noticed in soft tissues, as if a thin shell had separated from the outer layer of periosteal new bone.

According to Moghraby (1967) in eumycetoma osteolysis predominates and is localized. The osteogenesis is seen as thin rim around lacunae as "Weaver bird nest appearance". Thus the bone reaction takes the form of rounded and clearly inscribed defects or cavities due to localized solid masses of grains gradually replacing the osseous tissue and marrow whereas in actinomycotic mycetoma bone destruction is more marked and assumes a reticular pattern due to osteolysis admixed with periosteal reaction having comparatively more osteogenesis. The affected bone may be thickened as fresh lamellae deposited beneath the active periosteum.

Singh (1979) studied 262 mycetoma cases radiologically and found that 27.1% cases had bone involvement secondary to soft tissue involvement. Both destructive and productive changes in bone were observed in the form of cavitation, periosteal reaction and new bone formation. Productive changes in the form of periosteal hypertrophic reaction was seen in few cases and sequestrum formation was not seen.

Desai et al (1970) also noticed more or less similar radiological finding with increased space between affected bone due to soft tissue invasion.

Table 1: Radiological study of Mycetoma (Sharma et al 1990).

Radiological characteristics	Eumycetoma	Actinomycotic mycetoma
1. Bone involvement	Localized	Diffuse
2. Periosteal reaction	Linear	Spicular
3. Patchy absorption of bone	Present	Present
4. Erosion of bone	Present (+) cavitation more marked	Present (+)
5. Medullary sclerosis	May or may not be present	Present
6. Osteolytic lesions	Usually present	Not so
7. Increased interosseous distance, subluxation of joint, calcification of ligament and even of disc	Usually not present	Present

Sharma et al (1990) performed radiological study on 303 cases of mycetoma, which included both eumycetoma and actinomycotic mycetoma cases. They found that bone involvement was present in 57.7% cases of eumycetoma and 75.8% cases of actinomycotic mycetoma. There was characteristic differences in the radiological appearance of bone lesions in two types of mycetoma. The periosteal reaction was found to be linear type in eumycetoma while it was spicular type in actinomycotic mycetoma. Bone erosion was present in both types. The cavitation of bones was more marked in eumycetoma. Depending upon the extent of periosteal reaction and destruction of bone, there was thickening or thinning of respective bone. When thinning occurred inter-metatarsal space widened which was seen in either type of mycetoma but it was more marked in cases of actinomycotic mycetoma. Sequestration and ankylosis were not so common. Osteoporosis was seen in both types of mycetoma. In actinomycotic mycetoma of spine, there was calcification of intervertebral ligment and discs. Sharma et al (1990) concluded that there were more osseous involvement and destructive lesions in actinomycotic mycetoma.

Delahaye et al (1962), Davis (1958), Destombes et al (1958), Vanbreuseghem (1958), Desai et al (1970), Singh (1979), Sharma et al (1990) have made remarkable studies in the diagnosis of species of mycetoma from radiological appearance. Vanbreuseghem (1958) and

Delahaye et al (1962) observed that extent of bone damage vary with different species and increasing in order with *A. madurae*, *M. mycetomatis*, *S. somaliensis* and the most destructive of all being with *A. pelletieri*. The size of bone cavities may be helpful in judging the nature of the organisms (Desai et al 1970; Singh 1979; Fahal and Hassan 1992). Large and few cavities are suggestive of *M. mycetomatis*, large multiple cavities with minimum destruction denotes *A. madurae* infection, large number of small cavities with extensive fuzzy destruction of bones are due to *A pellitieri* or *S. somaliensis* infection. Extensive bone destruction without cavitation is suggestive of *N. asteroides* infection (Desai et al 1970).

Singh (1979) observed that in *A madurae* infection there was massive destruction with multiple large and small bone cavity formation and limited destruction was seen with *S. somaliensis* infection which is contrary to the finding of Desai et al (1970). Cockshott (1968), Mahgaub (1968) and Crockett (1968) had also found extensive bone destruction with A pellitieri and *N. brasiliensis*.

Singh (1979) observed primary osseous lesion of mycetoma in 3.05% of cases studied. However, these intra-osseous lesions could only be diagnosed during operation or on histological examination. So far, the accetable theory which explain primary intra-osseous lesions is that of Cockshott (1961) who believed that infective agent is directly implanted into bone by thorn prick. This theory seems to be without much foundation, that thorn passing through the soft tissue does not leave a trace of fungus there and secondarily it is unlikely that a thorn can prick the cortex of cancellous bone directly. Apart from this, thorns has not been seen in bony lesions. Haematogenous spread had been documented by Kulowaski and Stovall (1947) and Abbott (1956) but this type of spread should lead to multiple metastatic lesions. On the contrary, Singh (1979) observed only solitary lesions. He found that all lesions reported in his study and previous studies were present in subcutaneous bones. As such soft tissue on the subcutaneous bones is very scarce and that too is firmly fixed to underlying bone and as no loose tissue is available for the growth of fungus, the latter from this focus directly invades the bone. This hypothesis is further supported by the fact that thorns were seen in the three cases in soft tissue adjacent to the bony lesion.

Philippon et al (1992) observed that patients with bone involvement were older (above 38 years) than other (below 28 years) and there was statistically significant relation between spontaneous pain and bone involvement.

Sharif et al (1991) compared use of M.R, imaging with C.T. scan. C.T. scan of lesions detects early bone changes and M.R. imaging detects precise extent of the lesions in the soft tissue both techniques are thus useful in management of patients of mycetoma. The characteristic "Weaver bird nest appearance" can occasionally be observed in C.T. Scan of mycetoma lesion. Braga et al (1993) had given emphasis on the use of bone and gallium scintigraphy for therapy and follow up of the cases of mycetoma.

Sonography of mycetoma may be of diagnostic significance as revealed by study published in Sudan. In eumycetoma the grains produces numerous sharp hyper-reflective echoes with no acoustic enhancement. Although the findings are similar in actinomycotic mycetoma but these hyper-reflective echoes are fine and settled at the bottom of cavities.

Chapter Eight

Pathology of Mycetoma

The characteristic macroscopic features of mycetoma are swelling, sinuses and grains (Abbott 1956, Lynch 1964, Conant et al 1971, Emmon et al 1977, McElroy et al 1992). Certain differences in morbid anatomy of maduromycetoma and actinomycotic mycetoma do exist. In early stages of maduromycetoma, lesions are well circumscribed and fairly localized within a fibrous wall. The lesion tends to follow fascial planes in its lateral and deep spread. In case of actinomycotic mycetoma, the extent of the lesion is often greater than the external appearance of lesion. The swelling has ill defined margins and it merges with the surrounding tissue. It is softer in consistency than that of maduromycetoma. The infection looks more bacterial than fungal. The cavities containing grains in both types of mycetoma are interconnected through the canals and communicated to the exterior (Mahgoub and Murray 1973).

The black fungal grains of *M. mycetomatis* tends to agglomerates in abscesses or encapsulated in fibrous tissue whereas in actinomycotic mycetoma the grains are yellow, red or white or non pigmented, tends to be single or multiple and scattered through out the tissues.

Histology of Mycetcma grains

The histological identification of various species of fungi causing mycetoma is easy and commonly employed method which has been emphasised in many studies (Mackinnon et al 1956, Destombes and Segretain 1962; Lynch 1964; Winslow and Steen 1964; Verghese and Klokke 1966; Chouhan and Agarwal 1969; Desai et al 1970; Koshi et al 1972; Reddy 1972; Sran and

Joshi 1972; Mahgoub and Murray 1973; Emmon and co-workers 1977; Joshi et al 1980, 1985, 1987; Sharma et al 1988, 1990, Venugopal and Venugopal 1991, 1995; Philippon et al 1992; Wanke et al 1992; Machado et al 1992; Alteras et al 1992; Fahal et al 1994; Mathur et al 1979, 1993, 1994; Singhvi et al 1995 and Sakand et al 1998). For histopathological diagnosis character of grains and surrounding tissue reactions are considered. However, it must be stressed that the histological appearance of grain establishes the diagnosis and not the tissue reaction which in most cases is not specific to the type of fungi. Generally, Haematoxylin and Eosin (H.E) stain is sufficient for species identification. In some cases of actinomycotic mycetoma, Gram staining and Ziehl Neelsen's staining are needed while in some cases of true fungal infections Gomori's methanamine silver staining, Periodic Acid Schiff (PAS) staining or Gridley's fungus stain may be necessary for bringing out the detailed fungal structure of the grains clearly. The histological description for both the grains and tissue reaction for different aetiological agents of mycetoma are as below -

HISTOPATHOLOGY OF EUMYCETOMA

Madurella mycetomatis

A). H.E. Stain - This fungus shows large 2-4 mm sized dark brown or black, bilobed or even trilobed grains which may be single or multiple and fragmented and cracked at places. The grain is embedded in brown matrix called cementing substance. The cementing substance is reddish brown to dark brown in colour, granular and abundant. This pigment is more prominent in the periphery than at the centre. Each grain consists of two parts medulla and cortex.

Two types of grains are produced by *M. mycetomatis*, a common one composed of relatively thin hyphae termed as filamentous type and a less common is vesicular type. The hyphae have radial or interlacing arrangement in longitudinal and transverse sections. The hyphae are large, segmented and contain round or oval chlamydospores which are both terminal and intercalary. Hyphae tends to be swollen towards periphery of the grain. Chlamydospores have thick walls and may be light eosinophilic or may even appear as empty objects devoid of any stain or some have brown pigmentation . In the less common vesicular variety, the whole grain is composed of large cells with peripheral localization of its brown cement around hyaline hyphae and chlamydospores.

Tissue reaction - The tissue reaction reveals a central area of suppuration with in which the fungal grain in present. The tissue reaction is variable. At places just around the fungus, it is predominantly neutrophilic. A little away from fungus, pigment ladden macrophages along with epithelioid cells are present. Micro abscesses with or without small fungal fragments are seen. In some areas, many foreign body giant cells admixed with pigment laden cells are seen depending upon the duration of illness. Varying degree of fibrosis may be seen.

Fahal et al (1995) studied host tissue reaction to *Madurella mycetomatis* and set new classification. They described three types of tissue reaction to mycetoma grains. Type 1 reaction is characterised by adherence of neutrophils to the surface of grain leading to its disintegration. In type II reaction, the fragmented grains and the dead neutrophils are cleared by macrophages and multinucleated giant cells while in Type III reaction, there is a discrete well developed epithelioid granuloma with Langhan's giant cells. The three types of reaction are usually seen in different combinations in same lesion.

(B). P.A.S. Stain- The fungal grain of *M. mycetomatis* is PAS positive. PAS positivity could be seen within the brownish hyphae. The neutrophils and macrophages contain pigment and PAS positive material. In PAS stained section, the cell wall of spores and hyphae stained bright pink, while cytoplasm appears less well stained. The spores and hyphae at the periphery of grain appeared pink while in the middle of the grain, they are either faintly pink or relatively unstained.

(C). G.M. Silver stain - With *Gomori's methenamine Silver staining*, the wall of the mycelium is stained dark brown to black in different area, thus sharply delineated. The spores are also stained dark brown to black. The cementing substance has similar staining. The background is stained pale green.

Madurella grisea

(A) H.E. Stain- In haematoxylin and eosin stained sections *M. grisea* exhibits approx. 1-2mm sized lobulated grains which are brown in colour and consist of two definite zones - a central non pigmented area made up of a loose tangle of hyphae without spores and interstitial cement and a dark coloured periphery composed of dense network of regularly arranged hyphae and round or polygonal structures embedded in brown pigment.

The whole grain has a hollow appearance due to the peripheral distribution of pigmented cement substance, this finding is contrast to *M. mycetomatis*, where the pigment is distributed uniformly in the grain.

Tissue reaction- The tissue reaction is predominantly mononuclear type. Just next to fungal grain clear space is usually present where neutrophils are abundant with no granulation tissue. Just little away from the fungal grain, neutrophils with large lipid containing cells macrophages, plasma cells as well as foreign body type gaint cells are present. The vascularity and fibrosis are insignificant.

(B) PAS Stain - The fungal grain is PAS positive In the peripheral area, the cell wall of spores, mycelial filaments and cement substance stains bright pink i.e. PAS positive whereas central area is weakly PAS positive or remains unstained in several cases.

(C) G.M. Silver stain- The Gomori's methenamine silver stain is positive for fungal grain. The periphery of grain is stained deep black. The mycelium and spores are quite distinct in this area. In central area of grain, spores and cement substance are not seen; only a few thin walled hyphae are seen thus giving it an empty appearance.

Phialophora jeanselmei or Exophiala jeanselmei

(A). H.E. Stain- In HE stained sections, the fungal grains are 1-2mm in diameter, irregular in shape and appear brown in colour. In section they appear as hollow spheres or as sinuous bands which sometimes called "vermiform" because of their serpentine form in thin section. The grain shows a dark brown peripheral zone usually surrounded by a narrow eosinophilic band. This zone comprises of mainly chlamydospores and few hyphal elements. The cementing substance is absent. The pigment is present in mycelium and spores. The centre of grain is non-pigmented devoid of fungal elements or contains a few indistinct hyphae. The pigmented curved fragile thin rind with central necrosis is characteristic of *E. jeanselmei.*

Tissue reaction- The tissue reaction is variable. At places just around the fungus it is predominantly neutrophilic. Centre of grain have inflammatory cells mainly consisting of polymorphonuclear leucocytes and lymphocytes. At places, around the small colonies, it is mononuclear, away towards periphery, the reaction is always mononuclear where foreign body giant cells and macrophages are predominantly present.

(B) PAS stain- Peripheral part of the grain is strongly PAS positive whereas central part takes faint PAS staining.

(C) GM Silver Stain- The fungal grain of Philophora is positive for GM silver stain. The spore walls takes distinctly positive black staining which make their appearance more distinct.

Leptosphaeria senegalensis

(A) H.E. Stain- The grains appears dark brownish black and about 400μm to1mm in diameter and found singly or in groups of 2 or 3. The border of grain is less even and is more crenated. The grains may be tubular or hollow with a pigmented periphery resembling those of *Exophiala jeanselmei* and *Pyrenochaeta romeroi*. The central zone of the grain is non pigmented and periphery is deeply pigmented. The grains may be smaller and otherwise they resemble *M. grisea*.

In peripheral zone, the wall of mycelium is having dark brown pigment and hyphae are irregularly arranged. The spores are numerous, large and prominent with dark brown cell wall and irregularly distributed in cement substance.

The central zone is devoid of pigment and cement substance. Mycelium in this part are numerous, segmented and may have bamboo stem appearance, with non pigmented wall. Spores are less in number and irregularly arranged.

Tissue reaction- The tissue reaction is predominently neutrophilic just around the fungus. Little away from the fungus, macrophages, plasma cells multinucleated foreign body giant cells are also present. The centre of grains usually have abscesses containing bacteria.

(B). PAS Stain- The PAS stain is positive for fungal grain. The mycelium in the peripheral part stains bright pink whereas central part of the grain stains light pink. The pigment and cement substance present in peripheral part are PAS positive.

Pyrenochaeta romeroi

The grains are soft and black which may be spherical or tubular or irregularly curved sheets of 0.5 to 1.5mm diameter resembling those of *M. grisea*. The grains are surrounded by a fringe of eosinophilic amorphous material. The brown colour of the cortex is derived from two layers of different degree of pigmentation. The grain is devoid of cement and has non-pigmented centre composed of hyphal elements. The grain is bordered by an eosinophilic band. Towards the periphery, the pigment increases in intensity and vesicles are present with double contour walls.

Allescheria boydii or Pseudallescheria boydii and Cephalosporium species

(A) H.E. Stain- In haematoxylin and eosin stained sections, no distinction can be made between the grains of A. boydii and those produced by Cephalosporium. The grains are white to yellowish and upto 2mm diameter. The grain composed of dense, net work of thin hyphae and may form larger hyphae (15-20μ) and spores or vesicles when they approaches periphery. Cementing substance is absent. The grain takes up eosin stain which is slightly deeper at periphery. Spores of P.boydii are of large size in comparison to spores of Cephalosporium.

Tissue reaction- The tissue reactions of both the fungi are predominantly neutrophilic. Just round fungus, no clear space is seen but neutrophils are abundant, next to it, macrophages, plasma cells and foreign body type of giant cells with chronic granulation tissue are seen.

(B) PAS Stain- Grains revealed a PAS positive periphery contrasted with pale centre. The spores are strongly PAS positive whereas mycelum filaments are weakly PAS positive.

(C) GM Silver Stain- The peripheral part of grains of *P. boydii* and *Cephalosporium* are black while centre is slightly black stained. The wall of mycelium are lightly stained whereas spores takes dark black stain.

Neotestudina rosatii

(A) H.E. Stain: Grains are white or brownish white, soft, more or less globose or polyhedral and 0.5 to 1mm in diameter. In section the grain is non-pigmented. A homogenous non-pigmented cement forms the outer border of the grain. Thin septate eosinophilic hyphae make up the outer third of the grain and they are embedded in the cement in a radial orientation, a characteristic which aids in the histologic identification of these white granules. Towards the centre, the hyphae become short, round and form vesicles of 6-15μm size which contains intracellular material. The surrounding tissue reaction is pyogranulomatous.

(B) PAS Stain: The fungal element is strongly PAS positive.

Aspergillus nidulans

(A) H.E. Stain- Grains are oval to round or bilobed measures 60-200 μm in diameter. The grains are seen in middle of micro abscesses. Hyphae are thin, faintly eosinophilic with pale spores distributed more towards periphery and surrounded by distinct zone of "Splendore-Hoeppli". The pigment and cementing substance are absent.

Tissue reaction- As the fungal grain is present in microabscesses, around grain there is a zone of neutrophils, little away from grain are present few macrophages, plasma cells and giant cells. Fibrosis is very little.

(B). PAS and GM silver Stain- The mycelium is PAS positive and take homogenous pink stain with PAS stain and with GM Silver stain mycelium stains light black.

Fusarium moniliforme

The grains of *Fusarium* are white. The grain is embedded in protenaceous material and surrounded by neutrophils and other inflammatory cells. Because the granules of this fungus are so similar to those of the *Acremonium spp.,* their differentiation without cultural studies would be very difficult. Curvularia geniculata and C lunata. It produces extensive tibrosis.

Curvularia geniculata and C.lunata

It produces black granule mycetoma in dogs identified histopathologically by granulomatous reaction around black grain with extensive fibrosis. The periphery of granule is composed of compact dematiaceous mycelium and chlamydospores which are embedded in a cement like material. The fungal elements towards the interior of granule are nonpigmented and consist of loose network of hollow thus resemble those of Leptospheria senegalensis.

HISTOPATHOLOGY OF ACTINOMYCOTIC MYCETOMA

Actinomadura madurae

HE Stain- The grains vary in size. They are round, multilobed with an irregular border. Two types of grains may be seen in the same section. A small grain composed of dense filaments staining homogenously and deeply with haematoxylin. A larger grain is having irregular margins with deep blue periphery. The centre takes a faint blue colour and it may be hollow. Both grains are surrounded by an eosinophilic zone which also varies in width. It increases with age of grain . It shows radiating filaments and clubs. Spores, pigment and cement substance are absent Mycelium are Gram positive.

Tissue reaction- Tissue reaction is mainly neutrophilic. Just around the grain a clear space is present and next to clear space, neutrophils are seen and granulation tissue is absent. Little away from the grain, neutrophils along with plasma cells and macrophages are present and giant cells are rarely seen.

Actinomadura pellitieri

HE Stain- Grains are red small about 60-150 microns in diameter. These are round, oval, lobulated or often semilunate may have an irregularly angulated border. The grain is deeply basophilic. Its border is sharply delimited without the fringe of hyphal tips which characterize the granule of A.madurae but many granules are bordered by a narrow eosinophilic zone. Mycelial elements are not easily seen. Spores and pigment are absent but cement like substance is present that stained dark blue or violet. The mycelium are Gram positive.

Tissue reaction- The tissue reaction is predominantly neutrophilic. Just around the grains are neutrophils in predominance and next to it are lymphocytes and macrophages. Fibrosis is absent with poor vascularity.

Nocardia species

It includes *N. brasiliensis*, *N. asteroides*, *N. caviae* and *N. transvalensis*. Species differentiation can not be made by the histological examination alone. Nocardia grains are white to yellow in colour, soft in consistency and round, oval or irregular with rounded edges.

(A). HE Stain- The grain stains eosinophilic with haematoxylin eosin stain. It consists of branched, segmented filaments with indistinct walls. The spore, pigmentation and cementing substance are absent. The periphery of grain is fringed, clubbed and surrounded by polymorphonuclear leucocytes.

Tissue reaction- Just around the fungal grain, clear space is absent, neutrophils are marked and granulation tissue is absent. Next to these cells a few macrophages and plasma cells may be seen. Giant cells are absent. Vascularity is of moderate degree and fibrosis is less prominent.

(B) Other stains - The Nocardial grains are negative for PAS and GM silver stain but these are strongly Gram positive showing branching filaments of variable length with in the matrix of the grain Nocardia grains are weakly acid fast with ZN staining.

Streptomyces somaliensis

(A) HE Stain- The grains appear round or oval or multilobed yellow to brown, smooth or hard and measured 0.5 to 1mm.and shows many longitudinal cracks. The grain takes light basophilic stain but it is eosinophilic towards periphery. The grain exhibit a smooth border without "clubs". The cement substance is abundant. Hyphal elements are seen as delicate faintly basophilic filaments in the cement. The pigment and spores are absent.

(B) Grams Stain: The grains of *S. somaliensis* shows Gram positive hyphae. In Gram stained sections, hyphal filaments at pheriphery are stained deep purple and these hyphae are separated by cementing substance which makes the grain hard.

Tissue reaction- It is predominantly neutrophilic just around the fungal grain a clear space is present along with a wide zone of neutrophilic infiltration. Next to it is admixture of neutrophils, macrophages and plasma cells and gaint cells. The gaint cells are foreign body and Langhans' type attempting to engulf the granule. A narrow zone of granulation tissue with poor vascularity and fibrosis are seen at periphery.

HISTOPATHOLOGY OF BOTRYOMYCOSIS

(A) HE Stain- The *Staphylococues* spp. and *Pseudomonas* spp. producing white to yellow grain. The lightly basophilic granule is surrounded by radiating clubs of deeply eosinophilic "Splendore-Hoeppli" material. The clubs are prominent in *Pseudomonas*. The botryomycotic granules closely resembles the granules seen in actinomycotic mycetomas and eumycetomas. The *Actino-bacillus lignieresi* causing actinobacilloses in the tongue of a cow. It produces comparatively irregular large granules which are basophilic and surrounded by eosinophilic material. All features of fungus like mycelia, spores, and pigmentation are totally absent.

(B) Gram Stain- Gram staining of the tissue section shows clumps of non-branching Gram positive or negative bacteria i.e. cocci, cocobacilli or bacilli.

Tissue reaction- The tissue reaction is purulent inflammatory type. Next to grain clear space is absent it is occupied predominantly by neutrophils. Next to it are neutrophils with few macrophages and plasma cells. Giant cells are absent. Granulation tissue, vascularity and fibrosis are also very poor.

PATHOLOGICAL CLASSIFICATION

According to Singh (1998) all specimen of mycetoma can be classified grossly and microscopically. Grossly the mycetoma lesions may be divided into six types depending upon macroscopic appearance as follows-

Type I - Well defined cystic mass without sinuses.

Type II - Localized diffuse soft tissue with ill defined margins with or without sinuses.

Type III - Infiltrative lesions involving both soft tissue and bones.

Type IV - Bony cystic or cavitatory lesions.

Type V - Extensive invasive lesions.

Type VI - Proliferative or pseudoepitheliomatous lesions involving skin and subcutaneous tissue.

Histologically mycetoma can be divided into five type depending upon tissue reaction (Singh 1998).

1. Acute inflammatory cellular response only.
2. Sub acute inflammatory type.
3. Chronic inflammatory cellular response.
4. Sclerotic or fibrotic type.
5. Thick fibrous capsule along with chronic inflammatry cell response.

FINE NEEDLE ASPIRATION CYTOLOGY IN MYCETOMA

Looking to the use of fine needle aspiration cytology (FNAC) for rapid diagnosis of various pathological conditions, FNAC has also been tried for diagnosis mycetoma by few worker (Bapat and Pandit 1991, El Hag et al 1996). Bapat and Pandit, (1991), used FNAC for diagnosis of actinomycotic mycetoma, and found presumptive results and suggested that definitive diagnosis of the aetiological agents can be made by culture. El Hag et al (1996) selected 14 patients with different types of mycetoma lesions and aspiration was collected from lesions. The smear was reviewed without knowing the type of mycetoma and findings were compared with histopathological examination. In mycetoma the causative agents have a distinct appearance on cytologic examination. They are surrounded and infilterated by neutrophils. In a background of polymorphs, other inflammatory cells like histiocytes, lymphocytes and plasma cells are also seen. This allow differentiation from artifact and inflammatory lesions caused by other bacterial and fungi .

EL Hage et al (1996) gave emphasis on the usefulness of FNAC. They also claimed that there is distinction between result of FNAC of eumycotic and actinomycotic lesions and they found that mycetoma can be accurately diagnosed by fine needle aspiration cytology and recommended the use of FNAC for routine diagnosis of mycetoma as it is simple, inexpensive, rapid and sensitive technique.

Chapter Nine

Mycology and Bacteriology of Mycetoma

Direct examination of discharge specimen from mycetoma lesions reveals presence of granules, which are characteristic of certain aetiological agents of mycetoma. The experienced investigators can identify certain species of fungus by examining the size, shape, colour and consistency of granules and knowing the agents prevalent in particular geographic area. However, final identification of organisms causing mycetoma can only be obtained by studying morphology and biochemical properties of pure culture.

Direct examination of granules is done in 10% NaOH or 10 to 40% KOH depending upon consistency of granules. The granules and few drops of KOH are taken over slide. The granules are crushed between slide and coverglass by gentle pressure. KOH mount is kept for few hours in moist chamber and examined under microscope specially to note hyphal dimensions, septation, pigment formation in hyphal walls, occurence of interhyphal cementing material, presence or absence of chlamydospores or spores. The consistency of granules and manner of its fragmentation are also noted. For stained preparation, the granules are crushed in pus in which it is found and films are prepared for Gram and Z.N. staining.

The grains are the prime source for culture. They must be alive and as free as possible from bacterial and fungal contaminations. Biopsy material is usually considered the best as it is good source of alive granules for culture, but if this is not possible, the grains extruded from sinuses may be collected. When eumycetoma is suspected washing of grains in sterile saline containing antibiotic is done to free them from tissues and bacteria. Many grains collected from sinuses may not be viable, but grains from centre of clean biopsy specimen are capable of giving a pure growth without any treatment.

The granules from suspected eumycetoma are inoculated on sabouraud's dextrose agar with antibiotics. Modified sabouraud's agar (2% glucose, 1 percent neopeptone, pH 6.5 to 7) is usually a satisfactory medium. Most of the fungi are sensitive to actidione therefore this antibiotic is never used in isolation of aetiological agents of mycetoma.

If direct examination shows Gram positive bacteria (Actinomycotic mycetoma) the grains are washed with sterile saline without antibiotics and inoculated on sabouraud's dextrose agar without antibiotics. Simultaneously blood agar, Lowenstein Jensen (LJ) medium and brain heart infusion agar are also inoculated.

As many grains as possible should be inoculated on to the medium, this is because only few grains may be viable which yield culture. Incubation should be done at 37°C and at 25°C because optimum temperature of the growth differs for different aetiological agents.

CAUSATIVE AGENTS OF EUMYCETOMA

Madurella mycetomatis

Our knowledge regarding *M. mycetomatis* is largely due to work of Mackinnon et al (1949a); Mackinnon (1951); Mackinnon and Vidal (1954); Mackinnon (1954); Borelli (1957) and Segretain (1958). *Madurella mycetomatis* was previously named as *Madurella mycetomi.* Its nomenclature was changed to M.mycetomatis by McGinnis (1980) as quoted by Machado et al (1992).

The grains are < 2mm, firm to brittle, oval to lobed, black hard, cemented together and have consistency to that of coal. A second variety of grain is also seen called vesicular or "open" grains having many large cysts. In KOH-mount preparation, the grains appear to consist of broad fungal hyphae, chlamydospores and cement material.

Colony characters: In culture, *M. mycetomatis* is extremely variable in rate of growth, morphological appearances and pigment production. The growth is better at 37°C than at room temperature. The colonies develop within few days as white mycelium which becomes greyish white to yellowish brown. A brown diffusible pigment appears in the medium making the reverse of medium dark brown. The colonies are smooth or folded, glabrous or powdery or leathery.

Black sclerotia may appear on the wall of the culture tube or deep in the agar of old culture in sugar free medium. Sclerotia consists of collections of dark round or polygonal cells. A needle mount of well-developed culture on sabouraud's, dextrose agar reveals broad, segmented, irregular hyphae from 2-6 μm and round chlamydospores measuring 5-15 μm. On corn meal agar, some strains produce short pointed conidiophores that bear flask shaped phialides with phialospores at their tips.

Rajendran et al (1991) evaluated straw-extract agar media for growth and sporulation of *Madurella mycetomatis* in comparision to conventional sabouraud's dextrose agar and soil extract agar. These media are made from wheat (*Triticum sativum*), Bajra (*Pennesetum typhoides*), Jawar (*Sarghum vulgare*) and Paddy (*Oryza sativum*). They used four types of straw-extract agar viz. Wheat straw extract agar, Bajra straw extract agar, Jawar straw extract agar and Paddy straw agar. Vegetative growth of *M. mycetomatis* on four types of straw extract agar was found to be superior to that obtained on the sabouraud's agar and soil extract agar. The isolates of *M. mycetomatis* sporulated better and faster than in conventional media. So Rajendran et al (1991) recommended straw extract agar as a sporulation media for *M. mycetomatis* and useful for studies of conidium ontogeny of the fungus.

Biochemical properties: *M. mycetomatis* assimilates glucose, maltose, lactose and galactose but not sucrose. It utilizes potassium nitrate ammonium sulphate, asparagine and urea. It hydrolyses starch. Gelatin is liquified and slight proteolytic activity is observed in serum or milk.

Madurella grisea

Mackinnon et al (1949b) identified *M. grisea* as new species of fungus producing black variety of maduromycosis in South America. Mackinnon and Vidal (1954) differentiated *M. mycetomatis* from *M. grisea*. Grains of *M. grisea* are black about 1mm in size. soft to firm in consistency, oval to folded, irregular with centre hyaline and periphery brown black.

Colony Characters: *M. grisea* grows better at 30°C than at 37°C. *M. grisea* colonies are 3 to 5 cm in diameter. These are rapidly growing, grey or olivarious and old colonies may become red-brown. The surface is somewhat cerebriform at centre and radially folded at periphery. The colonies are covered with short grey aerial hyphae.

Lactophenol mount made from the colonies shows septate, brownish black hyphae measuring 1-3 μm in diameter. Larger moniliform hyphae measuring 3-5 μm and chains of arthroconidia may also be seen.

Biochemical properties: *M. grisea* differs from *M. mycetomatis* in that it utilizes sucrose instead of lactose. Other properties are similar to that of *M. mycetomatis*.

Exophiala jeanselmei

This fungus was first isolated in 1928 from a case of black grained mycetoma of foot by Jeanselme on the island of Martinique (Jeanselme et al 1928). Langeron (1928) called this organism *Torula jeanselmei* because of the budding nature of conidia. Emmons (1945) transferred it to the genus Phialophora on the mode of conidiogenesis. However, Buckley and Murray (1966) suggested to bring it back to the genus Torula because there was no serological relation between *P. jeanselmei* and other members of the genus. After an extensive study by McGinnis and Padhye (1977), the organism was reclassified as *Exophiala jeanselmei*.

The granules of *E. jeanselmei* are brown and irregular in shape. Entire granule in pus sometimes appears as worm cast because of its elongated shape and irregular surface. In sections, the granules appear as hollow spheres or sinuous bands. The external surface is composed of brown, thick-walled hyphal tips and chalmydospore like cells, 4-8 μm in diameter. Towards centre, granules have smaller hyphal cells.

Colony Characters: The fungus grow well at 30°C producing raised or dome shaped colonies 2 to 2.5 cm in diameter in 2 weeks time on glucose neo-peptone agar. The colonies on sabouraud's dextrose agar are black and slimy. They become effuse, mycelial and covered with aerial hyphae. With prolonged growth, the colonies become velvety and lose its slimy appearance. Microscopic morphology reveals mycelium mat consisting of septate brown hyphae producing branched and unbranched phialides laterally or on the apex. The dimensions of the phialides are too variable. The simple tubular phialides are usually 1.5 to 3.5 μm in diameter and 5 to 15 μm in length. The branched phialides may be considerable longer. The spores or conidia are extruded from the tip of phialides. These are one-celled, subglobose, elliptical to cylindrical, smooth hyaline and aggregated in masses that tends to slide down the phialides or along hyphae in a microscopic slide mount.

Biochemical properties

All strains of *E. jeanselmei* assimilate glucose, maltose sucrose and galactose but not lactose. Assimilation of potassium nitrate is variable. They produce urease and do not liquify gelatin.

Leptosphaeria senegalensis

It was identified as a new species causing mycetoma by Baylet, Camain and Segretain in 1959. Its grains are black and measure about 1mm diameter. The grains may be tubular or hollow with a pigmented periphery.

Colony Characters: The fungus grows well at 37°C, growth is slow at low temperature. It produces grey to brown colonies. The reverse side of colony is black and some strains produce rosy tint in the agar. The centre of the colony is dome-shaped which produces radiating filaments, the latter are white and become brownish as they grow old.

Microsocpic morphology of culture shows both fine and large hyphae. The mycelium is branched and slightly swollen at places. Arrangement of hyphae looks like the mesh of a net. Chlamydospores are rarely seen. On prolonged incubation i.e. for one to two months the fungus produces perithecia or ascocarps 100 to 300μ diameter. The asci are 17 to 22 x 80 to 110 μ in size and each contains 8 ascospores which are 8 to 10 x 23 to 30 μ in size. They are usually hyaline but may be brown. The ascospores are covered with a mucilagenous sheath.

El-Ani (1966) described a new species of *Leptosphaeria* known as *L. tompkinsii* on the basis of greater size of perithecium, asci and ascospores. Ascospores are narrower towards the end, more bent or curved than those of *L. senegalensis* and having a thinner mucilaginous sheath.

L. tompkinsii was also reported by Segretain in 1962 and Segretain et al in year 1974 in patients coming from Paris and Senegal. In India, this rare fungus was reported by Venugopal and Venugopal (1990b).

Biochemical properties: The fungus assimilates glucose, galactose, sucrose and maltose. Its growth is poor in presence of lactose.

Pyrenochaeta romeroi

The *P. romeroi* was first identified as new species causing maduromycetoma by Borelli (1959). *P. romeroi* produces soft black, spherical or tubular granules or irregularly curved sheet which varies in diameter 0.5 to 1.5mm.

Colony Characters: The organism grows well at around 30°C. In culture the colonies are dark grey, floccose with white periphery and black pigmentation visible on reverse side of colony. The fungus produces brownish-black ostiolate pycnidia 50 to 150 x 100 to 300 μ which bear elliptical pycnidiospores 1 to 1.3 x 2 to 5 μ. The granules of *P. romeroi* are similar to that of *M. grisea* and colonies of the two fungi are similar in culture. Some strains of *M. grisea* under suitable condition also produce masses which look like abortive pycnidia.

Allescheria boydii (Pseudallescheria boydii or Petriellidium boydii)

Allescheria boydii is the perfect stage of *Scedosporium apiospermum* (Emmon 1944 and Ajello 1952). It produces white to yellow, soft to firm, spherical or lobulated grains. Hyphae of the grain are hyaline and measures 2 to 5 μ in diameter. Large hyphae with diameter 15 to 20 μ are also present at periphery. Peripheral hyphal cells are large and modified in shape and size by environment present in tissue.

Colony characters: In culture, the growth is cottony, 'fluffy' and white initially later its centre turns brown and periphery of growth becomes greyish white. The reverse of colony is grey-white. The fungus grows well at 30°C to 37°C. Microscopically, septate hyphae with oval or club shaped pale brown conidia are seen. These conidia are borne singly or in groups on lateral or terminal conidiophores, varies in size from 3.5 to 7 x 5 to 12 μ in diameter, seen on the aerial hyphae at the edge of slant. Each ascus bear 8 ascospores. The ascospores are elliptical 4 to 5 x 7 to 8 μ with faint brown wall.

Biochemical properties: It assimilates glucose, but not maltose and lactose. Asparagine, potassum nitrate, ammonium sulphate and urea are assimilated by it. It has proteolytic activity for serum gelatin and milk.

Acremonium species (Cephalosporium Sp.)

Previously it was known as *Cephalosporium*. Various species of *Cephalosporium* viz. *C. falciforme*, *C. recifie* and *C. acremonium* may cause mycetoma. *C. granulomatis* is synonym of *C. acremonium* (Mackinnon 1954). *Cephalosporium* species produce pale white grains. These may be elongated and irregular.

Colony characters: On glucose pepone agar colonies are round and radially folded. The aerial mycelia are of lilac or light purple colour. A diffusible purple pigment is present in the medium. Microscopically septate hyphae are seen which produces unbranched tube like phialide. Conidia are present at the tips of these phialides to form spherical masses. These conidia are oval or elongated later becoming sickle shaped and one to two celled. Chlamydospores may be seen after two to three weeks of growth. They may be terminal, lateral or intercalary.

In case of *C. acremonium*, growth is better at 26°C instead at 37°C. Colonies becomes rose pink. Reverse side of colony is uncoloured, no diffusible pigment is present. (Murray and Holt 1964).

Biochemical properties: It assimilates glucose, maltose sucrose and galactose but not lactose. Urea, asparagine, potassium nitrate and ammonium phosphate are also assimilated. Starch is not hydrolysed.

Neotestudina rosatii

N. rosatii is a white grain mycetoma identified by Segretain and Destombes (1961). The grains are soft, globose 0.5 to 1mm diameter. Hyphae in the external layers of grain are narrow, septate and branched. Towards centre of grain vesicle like cells and few hyphae are seen.

Colony character: The growth is better at 30°C to 37°C. In culture mycelial mass is flattened or wrinkled covered with grey brown to white aerial hyphae. On corn meal agar it produces black spherical cleistothecia 350 μ in diameter. Its surface is surrounded by brown to hyaline hyphae and globose cells. Inside it are present asci containing 8 ascospores which are kideney shaped, two celled with thick brown walls.

Biochemical properties: Only lactose is poorly utilised.

Fusarium solani and F. moniliforme

It was reported to cause white grain mycetoma. In culture the colonies are flufty to cottony owing to extensive mycelia. Diffusible pink, purple or yellow pigment is produced on the reverse side of colonies. Microscopic examination shows conidiophores which are single or grouped into sporodocium, a compact mass of interwoven conidiophores. Conidia are produced singly or in groups are hyaline and unicellular or transversely septate. Macroconidia are cresent or bean shaped. Microconidia are single celled and found in chains or balls.

Curvularia species

C. geniculata and C. lunata have been reported to cause black grain mycetoma in dogs. (Elad et al 1991). On culture colonies are rapidly growing, floccose, brown with black reverse. Microscopy of the colony shows conidiophores which are simple bearing conidia apically from a new sympodial growth. The conidia are transversely septate and slightly curved.

Aspergillus nidulans

Following the first isolation of *A. nidulans* from a case of mycetoma in 1906 by Nicholle and Pinoy in Tunisia. No authentic report of mycetoma caused by this fungus appeared in literature until Baylet et al (1968). They reported its isolation from two cases of mycetoma of knee in Senegal. Later on other cases were being reported from other parts of the world.

The granules of A.nidulans are small 0.5 to 1mm, yellowish white in colour. Microscopic examination of crushed grains shows branching hyphae and spherical spores. On Sabouraud's agar, a whitish filamentous growth appears which turns light green on further incubation. Lactophenol preparation from growth reveals characteristic conidiophores with expanded terminal ends called vesicle having width of 8 to 10μ. Phialides arise from metulae which are attached to vesicle. Phialides produce long chanins of dark green coloured conidia of 3 to 3.5μ diameter.

CAUSATIVE AGENTS OF ACTINOMYCOTIC MYCETOMA

The causative agents of actinomycotic mycetoma belong to a group of aerobic actinomycetes which includes members of genera *Actinomadura*, *Streptomyces* and *Nocardia*. They are gram positive filamentous bacteria. The development of mycelium with true branching, the production of aerial hyphae in culture and branched filamentous appearance in tissues are features which differentiate this group from related organisms such as *Mycobacteria*. *Nocardia* species are differentiated from other genera of Actinomycetes by their partial acid fast character on modified Z.N.staining.

Actinomadura madurae

This species was previously called *Nocardia madurae* or *Streptomyces madurae*. Lechevalier and Lechevalier (1970) reclassified this species into new genus as *Actinomadura madurae*.

Table 2: Physiological and Biochemical properties of fungi causing mycetoma

Properties	*M. mycetomatis*	*M. grisea*	*E. jeanselmei*	*L. senegalensis*	*P. romeroi*	*A. boydii*	*A. falciforme*	*N. rosatii*
Assimilation of Glucose	+	+	+	+	*	+	+	*
Maltose	+	+	+	+	*		+	*
Lactose	+	-	-	+	*	-		-+
Galactose	+	+	+	+	*	±	+	*
Sucrose	–	+	+	+	*	±	+	*
Potassium nitrate	+	+	±	+	*	+	+	*
Ammonium sulphate	+	+	+	*	*	+	+	*
Asparagine	+	+	*	+	*	+	+	*
Urea	+	+	+	*	*	+	+	*
Hydrolysis of starch	+	+	*	*	*	+	–	*
Proteolytic activity on :								
Inspissated serum	±	±	*	*	*	+	±	*
Milk	±	±	–	*	*	+	±	*
Gelatin liquifaction	+	±	–	*	*	+	±	*
Growth at :								
37°C	++	+	+	+	+	+	+	+
30°C	+	++	++	+	++	-+	++	+
Pigmant	Brown	± Brown	-	Pink brown	-	-	Liliac	-

+ Positive, ± Most strain positive or weak utilisation, * Not known, ± Poor or most strain negative, - Negative, Cited from Mahgub and Murray 1973 with slight modification.

The grains of this fungus are 1 to 5 mm and sometimes upto 10mm in diameter. These may be spherical or angular with a lobated surface, soft and can be easily crushed to turn into suspension of pasty consistency. The colour of grains is white or yellow and rarely pink. The border of grain is composed of long fringed hyphae.

Colony Characters

The organism grows better at 37°C than at 30°C. The colonies rapidly grow on Lowenstein Jensen medium and on Sabouraud's agar. The growth is white to yellow, pink or orange with a shiny, glabrous, waxy wrinkled surface. Microscopy of growth shows delicate branching hyphae o.5 to 1 μm in diameter and may occasionally bear spherical conidia. The hyphae are gram positive and non acid fast.

Biochemical Properties

Actinomadura madurae hydrolyses casein, hypoxanthine and tyrosine and it produces acid from cellobiose. It does not hydrolyses xanthine. *Actinomadura madurae* is sensitive to the action of lysozyme. Lysosomal resistance can be tested according to procedure adopted by Finegold and Baron (1986). The *Actinomadura* genera is also differentiated from *Nocardia* and *Streptomyces* by O.N.P.G. (O-nitrophenyl-beta-galactosidase) test. The O.N.P.G. test is positive for Nocardia and *Streptomyces* and negative *for Actinomadura.*

Actinomadura pelletieri

The organism was previously labeled as *Nocardia pelletieri* or *Streptomyces pelletieri.* Later on it was reclassified as *Actinomadura pelletieri* by Lechevalier and Lechevalier (1970). Grains produced in vivo are small 300 to 500 μ in diameter, oval to lobed and typically bright ruby red.

Colony Characters

The organism grows best at 37°C. The colonies are slow growing and appear either folded or wrinkled. The colour is red and surface is waxy on Sabouraud's agar and sometimes covered with short white aerial hyphae on Lowenstein's medium. Microscopic examination of colony reveals branched hyphae less than 1 μm in diameter which do not fragments, which are Gram positive and non-acid fast.

Table 3: Differentiation of selected Aerobic Actinomycetes

Organism	Acid from cellobiose	Hydrolysis of					Lysozyme resistance	ONPG Test
		Casein	Hypoxanthine	Tyrosine	Urea	Xanthine		
Actinomadura madurae	+	+	+	+	–	–	–	–
Actinomadura bellitien	–	+	+/-	+	–	–	–	–
Nocardia asteroids	–	–	–	–	+	–	+	+
Nocardia brasilensis	–	+	+	+	+	–	+	+
Nocardia caviae	–	–	+	+/-	+	+	+	+
Nacardia transvalensis	–	–	–	–	+	d	+	+
Streptomyces somaliensis	–	+	–	+	–	–	–	+

d – doubtful, Modified from McGinnis et al 1982.

Biochemical Properties

The organism is differentiated from *A. madurae* by its failure to produce acid from cellobiose. It hydrolyses casein, hypoxanthine and tyrosine like *A. madurae*.

Nocardia

Infection with *Nocardia* species give rise to small white to yellow grains measuring 0.5 to 1mm in diameter and soft in consistency. They are aerobes and can grow well at 28°C or 37°C. Although Nocardia can grow easily on Sabouraud's dextrose agar without antibiotic and on Lowenstein's Jensen medium but growth may be better on selective medium. Ayyar et al (1992) compared the efficacy of three media namely modified Thayer martin medium, McClung's carbon free broth with paraffin bait and paraffin agar in isolating *Nocardia* species from clinical specimens. They concluded that paraffin agar was found to be an inexpensive and selective medium for isolation of *Nocardia* species when compared with paraffin bait technique. Microscopic examination of colonies can be best studied on slide culture (Gordon and Smith 1955; and Proctor 1966) which is incubated in moist chamber for two weeks using malt agar, glucose asparagine or soil extract media. It can also be done by the hanging drop method or block cultures (Young and Hotchkiss, 1959).

(a) Nocardia brasiliensis

Granules from pus are irregularly spherical often lobulated and may vary from 0.3 to 0.7 mm size, white to yellow and soft. Direct microscopic examination of granules in 20% KOH mount shows thin and branched filaments. The granules are surrounded with distant peripheral 'clubs' of varying shape and size. In stained smear of granules, the filaments are gram positive and acid fast by Kinyouns method.

Colony character

Growth may appear early on blood agar. They grow on Sabouraud's agar without antibiotics and L.J. medium. The growth matures in 7-9 days. The colonies are heaped up, wrinkled, folded and white, yellow or orange in colour with a moist or chalky surface. Microscopic appearance of growth shows delicate branching filaments, less than 1 μm in diameter. The hyphae are straight and beaded and soemtime coiled or fragment into bacillary and coccoid forms.

Biochemical Properties

Nocardia brasiliensis hydrolyses casein, hypoxanthine, tyrosine and urea. It shows resistance to lysozyme and gives positive O.N.P.G. test. It is differentiated from *Actinomadura madurae* by failure to produce acid from cellobiose and by its resistance to lysozyme and positive ONPG test.

(b) Nocardia asteroides

Its granules are white to yellow, majority of its strains when stained with Ziehl Neelsen method shows weakly acid fast slender branching filaments or rods of varying lengths. Short filaments and even coccoid forms may be seen (Gordon and Mihm 1962).

Colony character

The colonies in slide culture are loosely filamentous with long branching interwining vegetative hyphae. Only few colonies show fragmentation of undisturbed vegetative hyphae. All strains show short to long and few to abundant aerial hyphae. The aerial hyphae of about 30% of culture segments and turn into chains of bead like spores (Mahagoub and Murray 1973).

Biochemical Properties

N. asteroides does not hydrolyses casein, hypoxanthine, xanthine and tyrosine. It only hydrolyses urea. Like *N. brasiliensis* it fails to produce acid from cellobiose and it is resistant to lysozyme and gives positive ONPG test.

(c) Nocardia caviae

It was first isolated from ear of a guinea pig and named *N. otitidis* caviarum by Senijders (Emmons, 1977). The grains are similar to *N. brasiliensis*. According to Gordon and Mihm (1962) most strains show long tangled branching filaments and few may show rods as well. Acidfastness is apparent in some strains.

Colony characters

The colonies are glabrous, waxy, heaped-up, wrinkled and cream to peach colour on Bennet's agar. Tuft of short aerial mycelia are seen on Sabouraud's agar and the colonies may appear yellow to orange. The microscopy of colony reveals long tangled branching filaments and some strains show rods as well. Occasionally chains of bead like spores may form.

Biochemical Properties

N. caviae differs from *N. asteroides* by its ability to decompose hypoxanthine and xanthine. It differs from *N. brasiliensis* by its ability to decompose xanthine not casein and tyrosin.

Streptomyces somaliensis

The grains are spherical or lobulate, large up to 2mm size, yellow to brown, smooth and hard. When granules are crushed between slides they may break into angular fragments. Gram staining of granules shows gram positive hyphae and a cementing substance which makes grain hard.

Colony characters

Unlike *Nocardia* species the optimum temperature for growth is 37°C. It grows aerobically on solid media like Sabouraud's or Nutrient agar. They may grow on L.J. medium. Sectoring of colonies is common giving areas of varing consistency and mottled colonising areas of brown colour. The underside may show a yellow colour. Tufts of brownish aerial filaments develop which may become grey with time. The organism usually is non fragmented but may produce arthroconidia in chains. Gram staining of smear shows delicate branching filaments 0.5 to 1μm in diameter. They are non-acid fast (Chander 1996).

Biochemical Properties:

Like *Nocardia* species, S.somaliensis gives positive ONPG test but it differs from *Nocardia* by its sensitivity to lysozyme. It is differentiated from *Actinomadura madurae* by its failure to ferment cellobiose and positive ONPG test.

Chapter Ten

Serology of Mycetoma

There is no established procedure for serodiagnosis or assessing the prognosis of mycetoma. The immunological response of an individual with mycetomas has been assessed by several serological procedures such as complement fixation test, agglutination test, immunodiffusion test, counter immunoelectrophoresis, immunofluorescent antibody test, enzyme linked immunosorbent assay, western blot test and skin test. The skin test has not been diagnostically useful but serodiagnostic tests may be of great clinical significans. These tests can aid to diagnosis in two ways, not only they detect the presence of mycetoma but also differentiate various aetiological agents. Serological tests may of great help in identification and classification of various organisms.

In 1913 Claypole tried to make use of complement fixation test to establish relation between *Nocardia, Streptomyces* and *Mycobacterium tuberculosis*. The complement fixation test was also used by Nelson and Henrici (1922) to study sera from rabbits artificially immunised with *Streptomyces madurae* (A.madurae) and other *Actinomyces* species. Results of both the studies were nonspecific and there was cross reactivity amongst the groups.

Ultrasonic disintegration of mycelial filaments of *Nocardia madurae* and *Nocardia asteroides* was done for the first time by Ludwing and Hutchinson (1949) to carry out detailed study of agglutination and precipitation tests. These serological tests were also studied by Schneidau and Shaffer (1960), Gonzalez Ochoa and Vazquez Hoyos (1953) and Bevis (1961) and Zamora et al (1962). Gonzalez Ochoa and Baranda (1953) prepared carbohydrate antigen from *Nocardia brasiliensis* which proved to be specific when used as a skin test reagent in patient of mycetoma caused by *Nocardia brasiliensis*. Murray and Moghraby (1964) tried carbohydrate antigen and culture filtrate prepared from *M. mycetomi* (*M. mycetomatis*), *S. somaliensis* and *A. pelletieri* into the anterior surfaces of the forearms of patients of actinomycotic and maduro mycetoma. The patients with maduromycotic mycetoma failed to react to any of the antigen or reacted only to antigen derived from *M. mycetomi* (*M. mycetomatis*). The patients with actinomycotic mycetoma reacted to actinomycotic antigens. Similar work was done by Magnusson (1962) using Nocardial and Mycobacterial antigens on guineapigs sensitised by these organisms. Antigens made from *Nocardia* species (Bojalil and Magnusson 1963) and *Streptomyces* species (Mahgoub 1965) were tried as skin tests. The results of these tests were found to be variable. Mahgoub (1964) and Murray and Mahgoub (1968) used precipitation in agar gel by performing single and double diffusion techniques.

Jameson (1968) describe immuno-osmophoresis test in which antigen is run from a filter paper against patient's serum and a known positive control in slots in the agar. Precipitation line develops within 3 hours. This test was used for diagnosis of mycetoma caused by *Streptomyces somaliensis*.

Singhvi et al (1996) studied immunoglobulin profile i.e. IgG, IgM and IgA in mycetoma by radial immuno-diffusion method using tripartigen plates. All three classes of immunoglobulins showed increased concentration in cases of mycetoma caused by *M. mycetomatis* and *A. pelletieri*. The little rise in levels of IgG and IgM in mycetoma caused by *A .madurae* and *S. somaliensis* were seen, in those cases where there was bone involvement. IgA was consistently raised in all cases of mycetoma irrespective of causative agent and tissue involvment.

Salinas et al (1992) performed western blot analysis on 16 sera obtained from *N. brasiliensis* infected individuals by using various antigens seperated from crude extract of *N. brasiliensis*. They found that these patients always showed the recognition of six bands namely 61, 49, 45, 42, 26 and 24 kilodaltons (KDa). Sera from leprosy and tuberculosis patients reacted strongly with the 49, 45 and 42 KDa bands but weakly or not at all with 61, 26 and 24 KDa bands. Similar were the findings with sera from healthy control volunteers. Thus the three identified immunodominant antigens 61, 26 and 24 KDa may be of clinical value in the serodiagnosis of mycetoma. Salinas et al (1993) by using 26 and 24 KDa protein developed a conventional solid phase enzyme linked immunosorbent assay and tested serum samples from cases of mycetoma, tuberculosis group leprosy group and healthy individuals. They found that there was a close correlation between the clinical condition of the mycetoma patients and the anti-26 and anti-24 KDa protein antibody concentration and therefore they proposed the use of this assay in routine clinical laboratories to confirm the diagnosis of *N. brasiliensis* infection in human mycetoma cases. Wethered et al (1988) used enzyme linked immunosorbent assay for studying pathogenesis of mycetoma.

Boiron and Provost (1990) presented a western blot assay for the diagnosis of nocardiasis with a specific immunodominant 54 KDa antigen purified from a culture filtrate of *Nocardia asteroides* by immunoaffinity chromatography. The western blot technique was applied using antigen 54, 31 and 62 KDa to detect the immunologic response to *Nocardia.* Immuno detection was performed according to biotin-avidine system. They found that 54 KDa protein is a candidate to be used as a probe in the study of humoral immunological response to Nocardiae.

Salinas et al (1997) prepared monoclonal antibodies against P24 and P61 immunodominant antigens from *Nocardia brasiliensis.* They tried these monoclonal antibodies to locate the antigen in *N. brasiliensis* cells by immunofluorescence. The lack of reaction with intact cells suggested that P24 and P61 antigen are not exposed in the complete bacterial cell surface. They prepared *Nocardia brasiliensis* cell extract and purified its two immunodominant antigens by polyacrylamide gel electrophoresis. By using an immuno-electro transfer blot method (Western blotting), they demonstrated that these two purified proteins reacted strongly with serum from N.brasiliensis infected mycetoma patients.

Joshi and Singhvi (1988) tried immuno-fluroscence test for demonstration of antibodies against aetiological agents of mycetoma. They demonstrated that out of sera obtained from patients of mycetoma caused by *M. mycetomatis*, *S. somaliensis* and *A. madurae* (the common aetiological agents of mycetoma in Jodhpur) only the sera obtained from patients of mycetoma caused by M.mycetomatis (commonest aetiological agents) gave positive test when mycelial fragments of this fungus was used as antigen. This test may prove to be specific amongst the types of cases studied.

Chapter Eleven

Experimental Mycetoma in Animals

Mycetoma is a known clinical entity. Its geographical distribution, age and sex incidence, mode of infection, aetiological agents, clinical presentation and treatment have been described in literature, yet lot more are to be known about its pathogenesis and effective chemotherapeutic agents. For understanding the pathogenesis animal models are the best by which it is possible to study the development of disease at various stages, incubation period, how organisms are implanted, what factors favour establishment of lesion after implantation and to search the effective drugs / chemotherapeutic agents. Knowledge about pathogenesis of mycetoma is hampered due to lack of an effective model for eumycetomas although there are reported experimental models for actinomycetes infection such as Nocardiasis.

Several investigators have studied the pathogenicity of different Nocardia viz. *N. asteroides, N. caviae, N. transvalensis* and *N. brasiliensis* in laboratory mice by various routes (Mackinnon and Artagaveytia - Allende 1956; Gonzalez Ochoa and Sandoval 1960; Destombes et al 1961, Gonzalez Ochoa 1962, 1968, 1973; Kurup et al 1970; Mishra et al 1973;, Gonzalez Ochoa and Sandoval Vuellar 1976; Beaman et al 1980; Malik et al 1982; Unaogu et al 1990; and Salinas Carmona and Torres 1996).

Mackninnon and Artagaveytia Allende (1956) used *Nocardia brasiliensis* by intraperitoneal route for study of pathogenicity of mycetoma. They noticed abscesses and grains after three weeks around the pancreas, in the omentum and between the liver and diaphragm. They also produced grains in guineapig by intratesticular route. Similarly Gonzalez Ochoa and Sandoval (1960) and Gonzalez Ochoa (1962) demonstrated pathogenicity of soil strains of *N. brasiliensis* by producing lesions and grains after 20-30 days of intraperitoneal inoculation. Destombes et al (1961) also used intraperitoneal route for studing histopathology of experimentally produced grains of *N. asteroides* and N.brasiliensis. Malik et al (1982) compared pathogenicity of three species of *Nocardia* viz. N.caviae, N.asteroides and N.brasiliensis by intraperitoneal route and they found that N.asteroides and *N. caviae* were more virulent in comparison to *N. brasiliensis*. Their finding that all the three species of Nocardia were pathogenic to mice was similar to the finding of Kurup et al (1970) and Misra et al (1973). George et al (1961) and Mohapatra and Pine (1963) also observed that N.brasiliensis is less pathogenic in comparison to *N. caviae* and *N. asteroides*. Gonzalez Ochoa (1968, 1973) inoculated *N. brasiliensis* into the foot pad of albino mice and maintained animal at laboratory temperatrue and his experiment resulted in the production of typical progressive mycetoma with sinuses and grains formation and he found there was no tendency to cure spontaneously.

Nocardia transvalensis was investigated for its ability to cause mycetoma by Unaogu et al (1990) in the skin and foot pad of mice. They succeded in producing skin lesion similar to mycetoma and found that Freund's incomplete adjuvant appeared to assist in the development of mycetoma lesions. The infection manifested itself as palpable nodules under the skin which discharged white to cream coloured pus containing nocardial granules. The lesions in the skin necrotised while those of foot pad resulted in bone destruction.

Unaogu and Gugnani (1990) studied the pathogenicity of *Streptomyces griseus* for laboratory mice both by intraperitoneal and intravenous route. Although it is an aerobic actinomycetes regarded as saprophyte but was found to be virulent for laboratory mice. The lesions appeared as nodules containing granules of *Str. griseus*. The granules of Str.griseus in experimental infection in mice resembled those of *Str. somaliensis* in human infection. Gugnani and Unaogu (1991) investigated the ability of Str.grisus to cause experimental mycetoma in the skin and in the foot pads of mice. They found that lesions appeared as palpable subcutaneous nodules discharging pale yellow, cheesy pus and granules of *Str. griseus*. They observed that the nodular lesions later became odematous with bone destruction and ultimately fibrosis developed.

Few studies are available for the production of grain-containing lesions by true fungi like *Madurella mycetomatis* (Borelli 1957 and Murry et al 1960) and *Pseudallescheria boydii* (Schmitt et al 1962 and Vanbreuseghem and Bernaerts 1955). Borelli 1957 produced typical grains of *M. mycetomatis* by inoculating mice intraperitoneally with a mixed suspension of *M. mycetomatis* and *Blastomyces dermatidis* or *Histoplasma capsulatum.* Murray et al (1960) used killed *Mycobacterium tuberculosis* as an adjuvant to a suspension of living *M. mycetomatis* which was injected intraperitoneally. Granulomatous lesions appeared after 3-4 weeks that contained well formed characteristic black grains of M.mycetomatis. The lesions were commonly seen in the omentum adherent to spleen, stomach or liver. Schmitt et al (1962) produced pin-point lesions in the liver and spleen of mice by giving 2.8 x 10^3-10^4 viable cells of *Pseudallescheria boydii* intraperitoneally. Vanbreuseghem and Bernaerts (1955) inoculated *P. boydii* by intratesticular route in rats and guinea pigs and managed to produce grains of *P. boydii* in testis of one rat.

Chapter Twelve

Treatment of Mycetoma

Successful management of mycetoma is still a therapeutic problem. The treatment of mycetoma consists of two main therapeutic modalities which may be either surgical or medical or both. Actinomycotic mycetoma is more amenable to medical treatment and long term remission may be obtained by chemotherapeutic agents if taken for prolonged period whereas eumycetoma are relatively resistant to medical treatment which may be due to presence of cement like substance around the organisms of eumycetoma demonstrable by ultra-structural studies (Fahal and Hassan 1992).

MEDICAL TREATEMENT

Indication for medical treatment: Following are the indications for medical treatment:

1. Lesions belonging to actinomycotic mycetoma
2. Extensive lesions where even surgery fails to provide cure.
3. Infilterative and invasive lesions where amputation for radical cure has been refused.
4. As an adjunct to surgery in eumycetoma.
5. Extensive lesions where surgery can not be performed effectively owing to the particular site of lesion.

Various drugs have been claimed to be effective against aetiological agents of mycetoma both in vitro and in vivo. Drugs which are effective in vitro can be tried for cure of experimental mycetoma in animals and then these drugs may be considered for treatment of human cases.

Antibiotic sensitivity of actinomycotic mycetoma agents in vitro:

Mackinnon et al (1958) investigated inhibitory effect of chemotherapeutic agents in vitro against the causal organisms of actinomycotic mycetoma. They found Dapsone was effective against *N. brasiliensis, N. asteroides, S. somaliensis* and *S. madurae* (*A. madurae*). These organisms being inhibited by concentrations of 10-20μg/ml of the drug. S.pelletieri (A.pelletieri) was less susceptible (MIC=50 μg/ml). Sulphathiazole inhibited the growth of *N. asteroides* at concentrations of 5-10 μg/ml, *A. madurae* was more sensitive (12μg/ml) and higher concentration (50-200 μg/ml) of this drug was required for inhibition of growth of *S. somaliensis* and *A. pelletieri. S. somaliensis*, *A. madurae* and *A. pelletieri* were sensitive to Streptomycin, Aureomycin and Chloramphenicol but only S.somaliensis and A.pellitieri were found to be sensitive to Penicillin. Mariat and Satre (1961) carried out test in vitro with Sulphamethoxypyridazine. They found that growth of *A. madurae* was inhibited by 4-16 μg/ml of the drug, *N. brasiliensis* and *A. pelletieri* were inhibited by 8-16 μg/ml and *S. somaliensis* and *N. asteroides* by 64-256 μg/ml of the drug. Sebastaio et al (1956) tried Sulfisoxazole (gantrisin) 3,4-dimethyl 5-sulfanilamide isoxazole in vitro against *N. brasiliensis* and found that concentration of 1.5 to 6 mg per 100 ml inhibited growth of this organism.

Mahgoub (1976) performed in vitro drug sensitivity test for *S. somaliensis, A. madurae, A. pellitieri* and *N. brasiliensis*. Drugs used for antibacterial sensitivity were Dapsone, Sufamethoxazole-trimethoprim, Streptomycin, Sulfadoxine-pyrimethamine and Rifampicin alone or in combinations. It was noticed that Dapsone did not inhibited the growth of organisms below 100 μg/ml of the drug whereas Sulfamethoxazole-trimethoprim and Streptomycin were effective at 25 μg/ml. On the whole Sulfamethoxazole-trimethoprim inhibited more isolates than the other drugs. Large number of isolates were inhibited when drugs were used in combinations than alone.

Medical treatment of actinomycotic mycetoma

Clinical cure in actinomycotic mycetoma with medical treatment has been reported by various workers (Sebastaio et al 1956, Ziprkowsky et al 1957, Latapi 1960; Cockshott and Rankin 1960; Lavelle 1966; Mahgoub 1972 and 1976; Mahgoub and Murray 1973; Gugnani et al 1981; Bendle et al 1987;

Venugopal and Venugopal 1991; Wanke et al 1992; Castro et al 1993; Gomez et al 1993; Wortman et al 1993 and Welsh et al 1995).

Sebastaio et al (1956) tried Sulfisoxazole 3,4 dimethyl-5-sulfanilamide isoxazole in a daily dose of 20gm orally in *N. brasiliensis* infection. Clinical cure was obtained after 2 months of treatment. Ziprkowsky et al in 1957 treated mycetoma caused by *A. madurae* and *S. somaliensis* with Streptomycin. Latapi (1960) tried Griseofulvin in the treatment of eight cases of mycetoma caused by N.brasiliensis. Results were poor in two cases. Cocksholt and Rankin (1960) produced apparent cure in three cases of mycetoma caused by *N. brasiliensis* with preliminary course of wide spectrum antibiotic for checking secondary bacterial infection along with 100 mg of Dapsone twice daily for two years. Lavalle (1966) tried Dapsone and Sulphonamide combination in actinomycotic mycotic mycetoma caused by *N. brasiliensis* for successful treatment. Dapsone along with Fansil (R04-4393) and Septran (Sulphamethoxazole and trimethoprim) was tried in the treatment of 64 cases of actinomycotic mycetoma caused by *S. somaliensis*, *A. madurae* and *A. pellitieri*. Complete cure was attained in ten cases and marked clinical improvement was noticed in 21 cases. Little improvement was seen in 26 cases and no responce to treatment in seven cases (Mahgoub and Murray, 1973). Mahgoub (1976) treated 144 cases of actinomycotic mycetoma where 63.2% cases were cured. The treatment was given even when there was advanced bone and lymphatic involvement. As drug level achieved in diseased bone was less in comparison to healthy bone so longer duration of therapy was required. The most effective treatment was Dapsone plus Streptomycin sulfate or Sufamethoxazole-trimethoprim plus Streptomycin. Sulfadoxine-pyrimethamine plus Streptomycin or Rifampicin also gave good result. Gugnani et al (1981) treated five cases of mycetoma caused by *N. brasiliensis* by administering 100 mg Dapsone thrice a day for six to eight weeks and found good results. Bendle et al (1987) tried Streptomycin in combination with Sulfamethoxazole and trimethoprim or Dapsone as recommended by Mahgoub (1976) and noticed variable results. Venugopal and Venugopal (1991) also found that combination of Dapsone and Streptomycin was effective against actinomycotic mycetoma. Wanke et al (1992) failed to treat mycetoma caused by *A. madurae* by giving oral tetracycline for six months. This treatment did not improve patient clinically as well as radiologically but in another patient having similar aetiological agent oral Tetracycline and Sulfonamide brought discrete improvement.

Castro et al (1993) elected treatment consisting of combination of Sulfamethoxazole (800mg) and Trimethoprim (100 mg) with Prednisone (10mg) orally daily. Wortman (1993) added drug Amikacin, Amoxycillin and clavulanate to commonly used drug Sulfamethoxazole and trimethoprim for treatment of *Nocardia brasiliensis* mycetoma. Gomez et al (1993) made the use of Amoxycillin and clavulanic acid in two cases of mycetoma caused by *N. brasiliensis*. Both cases having bone involvement and these were resistant to the commonly used drug. The tablet containing 500 mg of Amoxycillin and 125 mg of Calvulonic acid was used. A dose of three tablets a day for 5-6 months was given. Gomez et al (1993) proposed this antibiotic as a new option for the treatment of some special cases of actinomycotic mycetoma with bone or visceral involvement or resistance to the drugs commonly used in this disease. According to Welsh et al (1995) treatment of choice of actinomycotic mycetoma is Trimethoprim-sulfamethoxazole alone or together with diamino-diphenyl sulfone. Amikacin can be used for severe cases unresponsive to previous treatment.

Antimycotic sensitivity of eumycetoma agents in vitro

Antimycotic sensitivity of eumycetoma agents in vitro revealed sensitivity to few drugs. Abbott (1956) tested antibiotics like Chlorampheniol, Oxytetracyclin, Carbomycin and Polymyxin B for in vitro sensitivity against the growth some of agents of eumycetoma. He found that growth of the M.mycetomatis was uneffected whereas *S. somaliensis* was markedly inhibited to all these antibiotics used. The growth of *M. mycetomatis* and *L. senegalensis* can be inhibited by 1μg/ml of Amphotericin where as that of *A. boydii* and *C. falciforme* were partially inhibited by 100μg/ml. Griseofulvin inhibited the growth of M.mycetomatis in concentration between 5 and 50μg/ml in vitro but *M. grisea* and *L. senegalensis* were not affected at this concentration (Drouchet and Segretain 1960).

Murray and Colichon (1962) investigated effect of Amphotericin B, Griseofulvin, Cycloheximide and Diamidinodiphenylamine on *M. mycetomatis* in vitro and found that Diamidino-diphnylamine had maximum effect on growth of *M. mycetomatis*. They suggested that Diamidinodiphenylamine might be a useful adjuct to surgery. Mahgoub (1976) tested Clotrimazole on 33 and Griseofulvin on 15 isolates of M.mycetomatis. A concentration as low as 1μg/ml inhibited about 21% of the isolates and 82% of the isolates were inhibited by 10 μg/ml of Clotrimazole. In contrast Griseofulvin was weak and no isolate was inhibited at low concentration of the durg. However, 33% isolates were inhibited at 100μg/ml of the drug concentration. Venugopal and Venugopal (1993) tested antimycotic susceptibility of 17 strains of eumycetoma including *M.mycetomatis, M. grisea P. romeroi, E. jeanselmei* and *L. tompkinsii* against Ketaconzole, Itraconazole, Miconazole and Econazole by both microdilution and agar dilution methods. They found that Itraconazole and Ketaconazole were more active, inhibited 50% of the strains (MIC-50) at 0.5 and 1μg/ml and 90% (MIC-90) at 2.5 and 5μg/ml. The MIC 50s of Econazole and Miconazole were 2.5 and 5 μg/ml and MIC 90s was 10μg/ml for both the drugs. Zoutman et al (1991) showed the fungus *Cylindrocarpon destructans* which causes eumycetoma was sensitive to Amphotericin B and Ketaconazole in vitro.

Medical treatment of eumycetoma

Medical treatment in maduromycetoma has been disappointing as it is relatively resistant to chemotherapy in comparison to actinomycotic mycetoma. However, Neuhauser (1995) reported clinical improvement in a case of mycetoma due to *M. grisea* with Dapsone. Reiffercheid and Seeliger (1955) used Dioxydichlorodiphenyl sulphide in a case of mycetoma of the buttocks due to *A. boydii.* The mycetoma lesion was infilterated by injecting 0.5-1gm of the drug in oil at regular intervals of two to three days for several months. Mahgoub (1976) investigated the use of Griseofulvin plus Penicillin and Clotrimazole in mycetoma due to *M. mycetomatis*. The treatment with Griseofulvin (500mg three times daily) and Penicillin (6 to 8 lacs units daily) given for a longer period of time ranging from 1 to 10 years. Only two cases cured out of the twenty treated cases. Clotrimazole given orally or infilterated into the lesion failed to cure any of the case out of the 7 cases studied.

Mahgoub and Gumaa (1984), Alteras et al (1992) and Venugopal and Venugopal (1993) tried Ketaconazole in eumycetoma caused by M.mycetomatis with some success. Venugopal and Venugopal (1993) found some improvement after 8-24 months by giving Ketaconazole orally 400mg/day whereas Alteras et al (1992) noticed only partial response with the same drug. Bilusiak and Sviridiuk (1990) suggested use of Ketaconazole in adjuct to surgery. Baudraz et al (1992) claimed significant improvement with long term use of Ketaconazole in mycetoma caused by *Fusarium* species. Fincher et al (1991) recommended use of Amphotericin B. initially with addition of Ketaconazole or Fluconazole in later part of therapy.

According to Bayles (1991, 1992) Itraconazole has an impressive safty profile and enhanced efficacy can be obtained by combining Flucytosin and Itraconazole and given for prolonged period. Machado et al (1992) tried treatment of *M. grisea* infection by giving Itraconazole for 3 months without any significant improvement. Elade et al (1991) found good initial response with Itraconazole therapy in mycetoma caused by *Curvularia* but noticed recurrence when treatment was interrupted. Buiting et al (1993) performed curettage of fistulous ducts and adminstered Itraconazole and could observed only varied results. Degvari et al (1997) claimed successful treatment with four months course of Itraconazole in mycetoma caused by *Arthrographic kalrae*.

Subrahmanyam (1995) achieved high cure rate with administration of intra-arterial crystalline Penicillin 10 lac units at intervals of six hours via dorsalis pedis artery in cases of myectoma foot, but he has neither mentioned the causative organism nor the type wheather it was eumycetoma or actinomycotic mycetoma. But the point is worth consideration that he cured 19 cases out of 20 cases in whom intra-arterial chemotherapy was continued for 4 to 8 weeks. These results needs further confirmation.

Walker et al (1991) tried hyperbaric oxygen therapy in mycetoma of foot caused by *N. brasiliensis* in which both conventional management of surgery and antibiotic therapy was unsuccessful. The hyperbaric oxygen was administered in a recompression chamber (one hour of treatment at 1.8 atmospheres absolute followed by a 30 minutes ascento to surface pressure). A total 19 treatments were administered and successful healing of lesion was achieved.

Careful monitoring of haemoglobin level and white cells counts is essential while treating mycetoma patients because many drugs used in treatment may be capable of inhibiting bone marrow function e.g. prolonged treatment with Sulphamethoxazole trimethoprim or Dapsone (Mahgoub 1976). Treatment should be temporarily suspended when anaemia or leucopenia develops. The response of drug therapy is to be assessed by grades as described by Mahgoub (1976).

1. Cured (Grade A)
2. Greatly improved : All sinuses healed and swelling very much reduced (Grade B).
3. Improved : Most of the sinuses healed and swelling appreciably reduced (Grade C)
4. No change or deteriorated (Grade D)

The grading done for therapeutic response by Mahgoub (1976) does not included all criteria for improvement and cure, so following points must also be taken in addition to healing of sinuses and reduction in swelling size:

1 Reduction in pain and tenderness and discharge from sinuses.

2. Radiological improvement.
3. Skin over lesions start gaining normal texture
4. Follow-up biopsy shows remarkable change in histopathology. Grains should be disintegrated and take haematoxylin stain very faintly and when cure is complete whole granulomatous reaction should be replaced by fibrous tissue.

SURGICAL TREATMENT

Indication for surgery

1. All encapsulated lesions.
2. Localised superficial lesions where functional loss is minimum.
3. Case of eumycetoma which are relatively resistant to medical treatment.
4. Failure of medical treatment.
5. Recurrence following medical treatment.

The aim of the surgical treatment is complete excision of mycetoma lesion to achieve cure and this is not difficult so long as the lesion is small and localised. Surgical removal resulting in complete cure is possible only in 30% of patients (Fahal and Hassan 1992). Surgery should be performed under tourniquet at accessible sites to facilitate the identification of margins of swelling, as cutting through involved tissues leads to recurrence by transferring the fungal elements into other part of operation fields. The rate of recurrence after surgical treatment ranges from 20 to 90% (Sulttner et al 1990). Since actinomycotic mycetoma has illdefined margins a wide excision through healthy tissue should be the rule. In eumycetoma when the lesion is encapsulated great care must be taken not to rupture the capsule. Some authorities advise irrigation of wound with providine iodine at the end of operation to destroy any missed grains.

Approximately one quarter of all mycetoma cases requires amputation of part or whole of the foot and rarely, of hand (Lynch 1964). Radical removal of pathological focus and preservation of weight bearing surface of an extrimity should be aimed while performing operation. Medical therapy by Ketaconazole should be given prior to surgery (Bilusiak and Sviridiuk 1990). If mycetoma present at craniocephalic or vertebro-medullary sites with neurological manifestation then amputation is preferred (Badiane et al 1992). For avoiding the socially disatrous consequences of amputation a programme of extensive repeated excision of diseased tissue including bone may be carried out preferentially (Bendle et al 1987) Medical treatment before and or after surgery may be useful in certain circumstances (Welsh et al 1987; Bilusiak and Sviridiuk 1990; Witzig et al 1996). Witzig et al (1996) treated mycetoma of back due to *A. flavus* with decompressive laminectomy and fourteen months Itraconazole regimen.

Excision of affected part and administration of ciplin injection locally in upper extrimity of nocardial mycetoma has been tried by some workers and found encouraging result with healing of sinuses without recurrence. Similarly recurrence can be controlled by adminstration of solution comprises of carbolic acid (10ml), acetic acid (10ml) and glycerine (20ml) in 600 ml of water after surgery at local site of lesion. This solution have property of localising inflammation followed by fibrosis of part so as to minimise the chances of recurrence.

Singh (1998) carried out both medical and surgical treatment of 310 cases of mycetoma, and he failed to achieve cure even in single patient with only medical treatment. Singh (1998) laid down criteria in planning treatment and rendering advise to patients dependng upon clinical staging, modes of spread, pathological classification, tissue reaction and causative organisms of mycetoma as follows:

A. Clinical Staging:

Stage I and II: Lesions in these stages are curable if wide excision is carried out under tourniquet at accessible sites.

Stage III: It demands radical surgery for cure but no guarantee for recurrence.

Stage IV: These cases are not amenable to surgery. Palliation can be provided by currettage and drug therapy.

B. Modes of spread: According to Singh (1998) mode of spread also helps in planning the treatment.

(a) *Local spread:* Radical excisional surgery is advised.

(b) *Fascial plane spread:* Fascial plane spread can be precisely observed at the time of surgery by observing the granules at these site. But some times granules may not be nicely visible and this is likely to lead to incomplete excision. It is suggested that magnifying glasses should be used to observe the granules for determining the extent of lesion.

(c) *Spread along medullary cavity:* In this type of spread it is advocated that whenever a lower end of any long bone is involved, it should be sacrificed as a whole by disarticulation or higher amputation.

(d) *Lymph node spread:* In this type of spread cure is likely to be achieved by radical excision of primary lesion and metastatic glands.

(e) *Haematogenous spread:* It is a rare type of spread, all involved sites should be taken care by excisional surgery whenever possible.

(C) Pathological classification

(a) *Type I:* Mainly have localised cystic masses and remains stationary for years together without any distant spread. These lesions should always be excised as they provide best chance for cure.

(b) *Type II:* Localised diffuse lesions can also be excised under tourniquet with reasonable success rate.

(c) *Type III:* These are similar to clinical stage III and can be taken care by radical surgery.

(d) *Type IV:* These are primary bony lesions also demand radical surgery for cure, but temporary cure can be achieved in weight bearing bone by currettage and bone grafting. This method does not provide protection against metastasis.

(e) *Type V:* This type include extensive invasive lesions of perineum, scalp, back, thorax etc. and are difficult to manage and most often are fatal. Removal of diseased part as far as possible along with medical treatment is advised.

Tissue reaction

Singh (1998) advised that multiple biopsies should be taken from periphery of lesion to look for tissue response at periphery. If biopsy shows acute or subacute type of tissue reaction, it is likely that lesion is progressing faster and demand early amputation. If sclerosis is present it is unlikely that these lesions will progress fast and metastatise.

Singh (1998) advocated use of Grisiofluvin and Penicillin along with surgery for the treatment of eumycetoma. For the treatment of actinomycotic mycetoma he advised use of various drugs in combinations as follows:

a) Streptomethoxazole-trimethoprim plus Streptomycin

b) Sulfadoxine-pyrimethamine plus Rifampicin

c) Dapsone plus Streptomycin

In botryomycosis medical treatment is given based on the report of culture and sensitivity.

Thus it is evident that treatment of mycetoma can be rationalised based on status of swelling, regional lymphonde metastasis, mode of spread, gross pathological appearance of lesion, tissue response and identification of causative organisms.

References

1. Abbott PH: Mycetoma, a clinical and epidemiological study. Dissertation for the degree of M.D. Cambridge University, 1954.

2. Abbott PH : Mycetoma in Sudan. Trans R Soc Trop Med Hyg 50, 11-24, 1956.

3. Ajello L : The isolation of Allescheria boydii, an aetiological agent of mycetoma from soil. Am J Trop Med Hyg 1, 227-238, 1952.

4. Akagawa S, Hebisawa A, Shishido H, Tamura A, Watanable H, Sato K, Kurashima A, Mori M, Sagara Y, Fukushima K : Mycetoma forming pulmonary nocardiosis and endobronchial polypoid lesion. Nihon Kyobu Shikkan Gakkai Zasshi, 35(8), 878-882, 1997.

5. Aldridge J and Krik : Mycetoma of the orbit. Brit J Opth 24, 211, 1940.

6. Alteras I, Hagler J, Treatiner A, Morojinski G, Segal R, Sandbank M : Mycetoma with granules first case in a native of Israel. Hautarzi, 43(7), 446-447, 1992.

7. Anandi V, Jeya M, Subramaniyam C.S., Chidambaram N and Xavier TS : Actinomycotic mycetoma of thumb. Indian J Med Microbiol 15(1), 43-44, 1997.

8. Andleigh H.S.: Mycetoma foot-etiology and laboratory diagnosis. Indian J Med Sci 8, 631, 1954.

9. Ayyar S, Tendolkar U, Deodhar I. : A comparison of three media for isolation of Nocardia species from clinical specimens. J Post Grad Med 38(2), 70-72, 1992.

10. Badiane SB, Sakho Y, Ndiaye MM, Kane A, Kone S, Mauferon JB, Kabre A, Ba Mc, LY A, Gueye EM et al. : Mycetoma with neurological manifestations. Inherent therapeutic difficulties in these localisation. Dakar Med 37(2), 117-121, 1992.

11. Bapat KC and Pandit AA : Actinomycotic mycetoma, report of a case diagnosed by fine needle aspiration. Acta Cytol 35(6), 770-772, 1991.

12. Banerjee AK, Basu SP and Basu N. : Studies on mycetoma. Bull Cal Sch Trop Med Hyg 9, 113, 1961.

13. Basset A, Camain R et al. : Role des epines de mimosacees dans Iinnoculation des mycetomes (a propos. de deux observations). Bull Soc Pathol Exot 58, 22-24, 1965.

14. Basu N, Sanyal M and Thammayya A : Actinomycetoma due to Nocardia brasiliensis. Indian Med Gaz, 14, 257-262, 1974.

15. Bayles MA : Tropical mycoses. Med Klin 86, Suppl 1, 13-19, 1991.

16. Bayles MA : Tropical mycoses. Chemotherapy, 38, Suppl 1, 27-34, 1992.

17. Baylet J, Camain R and Segretain G : Identification des agents des maduromycoses du Senegal et de la Mauritanie. Bull Soc Path Exot, 52, 448-477, 1959.

18. Baylet R, Camain R, Bezs H and Rey M : Mycetoma - A Cephalosporium an Senegal. Bull Soc Path Exot, 54, 802-810, 1961.

19. Baylet R, Lacoste P, Camain R et al : Aspergillus nidulans agent of mycetoma. Bulletin de la Societe de pathologic Exotique, 61, 359-365, 1968.

20. Baudrauz RF, Monod M, Borradori L, Ginalsky JM, Vion B, Boccard C, Frenk E : Mycetoma of foot due to Fusarium species treated with oral ketaconazole. Dermatology. 184(4), 303-305, 1992.

21. Baxter M, Murray IG and Tayler JJ : A case of mycetoma with serological diagnosis of Allescheria boydii. Sabouraudia, 5, 138-140, 1966.

22. Beaman BL, Maslan S, Scales S and Roesen J : Effect of route of inoculation on host resistance to Nocardia. Infec and Immun 28, 185-189, 1980.

23. Bedi TR, Kaur S and Kumar B. : Red grain mycetoma of scalp (A pelletieri) A case report from India. Mycopathologia, 63, 127-128, 1978.

24. Bendle BJ, Mackey D, Al-Saati F, Sheth KV, Ofole SN and Bailey TM. : Mycetoma in Saudi Arabia. J. Trop Med. Hyg 90, 51-59, 1987.

25. Bevis ML. : Serological studies on Mycobacteria, Nocardia, Actinomyces and Fungi. Sabouraudia 1, 154-160, 1961.

26. Bidie G : Notes on Morbus Pedis Entophyticus, Madras QJ Med Sci, 4, 222-227, 1862.

27. Bilusiak DM and Sviridiuk VZ : Mycetoma, Klin Khir 1, 26-29, 1990.

28. Bocarro JE : An analysis of one hundred cases of mycetoma. Lancet 2, 797-798, 1893.

29. Bocarro JE : Clinical notes on mycetoma differentiating the pale from the black variety. Indian Med Gaz 29, 451-452, 1894.

30. Bocarro JE : On mycetoma. Trans Bombay Med Congress, 324-332, 1909.

31. Boiron P and Provost F : Use of partially purified 54 kilodalton antigen for diagnosis of nocardiosis by western blot assay. J Clin Microbiol, 28(2), 328-331, 1990.

32. Bojalil LE and Magnusson M. : Specificity of skin reactions of human Nocardia sensitins. Am Rev Resp Disease 88, 409-411, 1963.

33. Borelli D : Madurella mycetomi fialides fialospores inoculational raton. Boln Lab Clin 2, 1-15, 1957.

34. Borelli D : Pyrenochaeta romeroi n sp. Rev Dermat Venezolana 1, 1-3, 1959.

35. Boyce R and Surveyor N : Upon the existence of more than one fungus in madura disease (mycetoma). Phylos Trans R Soc Lond 185, Part 1, 1-14, 1894.

36. Braga FJ, Araujo EB, Cambrgo EE, Rivitti MC, Cuce LC : Scintigraphic evaluation of mycetoma. Nucl Med Commun 14(9) 814-818, 1993.

37. Bristowe JS : Fungus-foot of India, Report on Dr Fox's Madura foot. Trans Path Soc Land 22, 320-326, 1871.

38. Brounst G, Nakib A and Mariat F : Sur le premier cas de mycetome a Nocardia asteroides observe all Liban. Bull Soc Path Exot, 55, 964-967, 1962.

39. Brumpt E : Les mycetoma. Archs Parasit, 10, 489-564, 1906.

40. Buckey HR and Murray IG : Precipitating antibodies in chromomycosis. Sabouraudia, 5, 78-80, 1966.

41. Buiting AG, Visser LG, Barge RM and Vantwout JM : Mycetoma of foot, a disease from tropics. Ned Tijdschr Geneeskd, 24, 137(30) 1513-1515, 1993.

42. Cameron HM, Gatei D, Bremner AD : The deep mycoses of Kenya, a histopathological study in mycetoma. East Afr Med J 50, 382-395, 1973.

43. Carter HV : On mycetoma or the fungus disease of India including notes of recent cases and new observations on the structure etc of the entophytic growth. Trans Med Phys Soc Bombay 7, 206-221, 1860 (Quoted by Ghosh et al , 1950).

44. Carter HV : On mycetoma or fungus disease of India J & A Churchill, London, 1874.

45. Castro LG, Belda Jr W, Salebian A, Cuee LC : Mycetoma a retrospective study of 41 cases seen in Brazil. Mycoses 36(3-4), 89-95, 1993.

46. Chabra HL and Chugh TD : Mycetoma in the perineum. Indian J. Pathol Microbiol 19(1) 71-74, 1976.

47. Chadfield HW : Mycetoma of the foot. Mycopath Mycol Appl, 24, 130-136, 1964.

48. Chander J : Mycetoma, In Text book of Medical Mycology Imprint Publication, Page 83, 1996.

49. Changani DL, Pandhi SC, Popli SP and Joshi KR : Mycetoma of middle ear cleff J. Laryngol and Otol, 86, 651-656, 1972.

50. Chakrabarti A and Singh K. Mycetoma in Chandigarh and surrounding areas. Indian J Med Microbiol 16(2), 64-65, 1998.

51. Chalmers AJ and Christopherson JB : A Sudanese Actinomycosis. Ann Trop Med 10, 224-282, 1916.

52. Chalmers AJ and Archibald RG : The classification of mycetoma. J Trop Med Hyg 21, 224-282, 1918.

53. Chouhan SS and Agarwal S : Histological diagnosis of mycetoma A clinical study of 24 cases. Indian J Med Res 57, 71-77, 1969.

54. Chugh TD : Mycetoma, Indian J Med Res 63, 1402, 1975.

55. Chugh TD, Arora DR, Sabherwal U and Chabra HK: Mycotema. Indian J. Med. Res. 63, 1408, 1975.

56. Clarke PRR : Mycetoma of the testis, Lancet, II, 1341, 1953.

57. Claypole EJ : On the classification of the Streptothrices particularly in their relation to bacteria. J Exp Med 17, 99-116, 1913.

58. Cockshott WP and Rankin AM : Medical treatment of mycetoma. Lancet II, 1112-1114, 1960.

59. Cockshott WP : Mycetoma in tropical radiology. Howard Middle Min William Heinman Ltd. London Page 38, 1961.

60. Cockshott WP : Radiological patterns of deep mycoses - systemic mycoses , A ciba foundation symposium. J and A Churchill Ltd. London page 113-125, 1968.

61. Colebrook L. Indian Army Medical Reports, 1846, Cited by Chouhan SS and Agarwal S. : Indian J Med Res 57, 71, 1966.

62. Conant NF, Smith DT, Baker RD and Callaway JL : Manual of clinical mycology WP Saunders Company London, Third Ed. 1971.

63. Cooray GH : Fungal infection in Ceylon. Ceylon Med J 7, 185-196, 1962.

64. Crockett DJ: Mycotema, Phycomycosis and Histoplasmosis companion to surgery in Africa. E & S. Livingstone Ltd. Edingnurgh and London. Pp 54-73, 1968.

65. Dasgupta LR, Sunder Raj T and Agarwal SC : Actinomycetes from mycetoma and other cases around Pondicherry. Indian J Med Res 62, 762, 1974.

66. Davis AGM : The bone changes in Madura Foot, observations on Uganda Africans. Radiology. 44, 897-908, 1958.

67. Degavri B, Joujoux JM, Dandurand M and Guillot B : First report of mycetoma caused by Arthrographics kalarae. J Am Acad Dermatol 37(2), 318-320, 1997.

68. de Hoog GS, Buiting A, Tan CS, Stroebel AB, Ketterings C, de Boer CJ, Naafs B, Brimicomb R, Nohlmans Paulssen MK, Fabius GT : Diagnostic problems with imported cases of mycetoma in the Netherland. Mycoses, 36, 81-87, 1993.

69. Delahaye RP, Destombes P and Moutounet J : Les aspects radiologiques des mycetomes. Ann Radiol (Paris) 5, 817, 1962.

70. Desai SC, Pardanani DS, Shreedevei N, Mehta RS : Studies on mycetoma. Indian J Surg 32, 427-447, 1970.

71. Destombes P, Andre M, Segretain G, Mariat F, Cambin R and Nazimoff O : Contribution a l'etude des mycetomes en Afrique francaise. Bull Soc Path Exot 51, 815-875, 1958.

72. Destombes P, Mariat F, Nazimoff O and Satre J. : A propos des mycetomes a Nocardia. Sabouraudia, 1, 161-172, 1961.

73. Destombes P and Segretain G : Les mycetomes fongiques caracters histologique et culturaux. Arch Inst Pasteur Tunis, 39, 273-290, 1962.

74. Destombes P, Mariat F, Rosatii L and Segretain G : Mycetoma in Somalia - conclusion of a study between 1959 and 1964, Acta Trop 34(4), 355-373, 1977.

75. Diamont RD, Bennet JE : Disseminated N.brasiliensis infection Archives. Internal Med. 131, 753, 1973.

76. Dravid MN, Venugopalan A, Bharadwaj RS, Nene SS : Mycetoma due to Nocardia caviae, a case report. Indian J Pathol Microbiol 34(1), 62-63, 1991.

77. Drouchet E and Segretain G : Sensibilite a griseofulvine et a amphotericine B des agents des mycetomes fongiques. Bull Soc Path Exol 53, 863-869, 1960.

78. Elad D, Orgad U, Yakobson B, Perl S, Golonb P, Trainin R, Tsur T, Shenkler S, Bor A : Eumycetoma caused by Curvularia lunata in a dog. Mycopathologia, 116(2), 113-118, 1991.

79. EL Ani AS : A new species of Leptosphaeria, Mycologia, 58, 406-411, 1966.

80. EL Hag IA, Fahal AH and Gasim ET : Fine needle cytology of mycetoma. Acta Cytol 40(3) 461-464, 1996.

81. Ellerbe DM, Parson DS and Cook DR : Botryomycosis - Improved therapy for a difficult infection. Int J Pediatr Otorhinolaryngol 118, 41, 363-369, 1997.

82. El-Mofti A, Iskander IO, Nanda N and Zaki SM : Madura foot in Egypt. Br. J. Derm, 77, 365-372, 1965.

83. Emmons CW : Allescheria boydii and Monosporium apiospermum. Mycologia, 36, 188-193, 1944.

84. Emmons CW: Phialophora jeanselmei Comb. N. form mycotema of hand. Arch Path. 39, 364-368, 1945.

85. Emmons CW, Binfort CH, Utz JP and Kwonchung KG : Medical Mycology, Third Ed. Henry Kimpton, London Pg 437, 1977.

86. Fahal AH and Hassan MA : Mycetoma. Br J Surg 79, 1138-1141, 1992.

87. Fahal AH, el Toum EA, el Hassan AM, Maghoub ES, Gumma SA. : A preliminary study on the ultra-structure of Actinomadurae pelletieri and its tissue reaction. J Med Vet Mycol 32(5), 343-348, 1994.

88. Fahal AH, el Toum EA, el Hassan AM, Mahgoub ES and Gumma SA : The host tissue reaction to Madurella mycetomatis - new classification. J Med Vet Mycol 33(1), 15-17, 1995.

89. Fincher RM, Fisher JF, Lovell RD, Newman CL. Espinel Ingroff A, Shadomy HJ. : Infection due to the fungus Acremonium (Cephalosporium). Medicine (Baltimore), 70(6), 398-409, 1991.

90. Findlay GH and Vismer HF : Black grain mycetoma - A study of chemistry formation and significance of tissue grain in Madurella mycetomatis infection. Br. J Dermatol 91, 297-303, 1987.

91. Findlay GH and Vismer HF : Botryomycosis - some African cases. Int J Dermatol 29(5), 340-344, 1990.

92. Finegold SM and Baron EJ : Lysosomal resistance test. In Bailey and Scott's Diagnostic Microbiology. CV Mosby company, page 495, 1986.

93. Flavial N : Micetoma actinomicosico de rodilla estudio clinocoy micologia. Prensa Med Argent 45, 2799-2802, 1958.

94. Frey D : Mycetoma of the scalp in an aboriginal child. Austr J Derm 17(2), 7-9, 1976.

95. Fukushire R and Mariat F. : Notes Sur un mycetoma a Nocardia caviae observe au Japan. Bull Soc Path Exot 58, 185-188, 1965.

96. Gammel JA : The etiology of maduromycosis with mycologic report on two new species observed in United states. Arch Derm Syph 15, 241-284, 1927.

97. Gardens VJ, Calle GV, Cortes AC and Retrepo AM. : Micetomas, presentation de dos nuevus casosy revision del tema. Antioquia Med 16, 117-132, 1966.

98. George-Lucillie K, Ajello L, McDurmoni C and Hosty TS : The identification of Nocardia asteroides and Nocardia brasiliensis. Amer Rev Resp Dis. 84, 337, 1961.

99. Ghos LM, Dey NC and Panja D : Madura foot (Mycetoma) Ind Med Gaz 85, 288, 1950.

100. Gill : Indian Army Medical Reports 1842, Quoted by Carter 1874 (Carter HV : Mycetoma and fungal disease of India, I & A Publisher, Churchill, London 1874).

101. Godfrey J : Diseases of foot not hitherto described. Lancet, I, 593-594, 1846.

102. Gokhalay BB, Padhya AA and Tirumalachar MJ : Madura foot in India caused by Madurella grisea. Sabouraudia, 6, 305, 1968.

103. Gomez A, Saul A, Bonifaz A, Lopez A : Amoxicillin and Calvulanic acid in the treatment of actinomycetoma. Int J Dermatol 32(3), 218-220, 1993.

104. Gonzalez -Ochoa A and Vazquez-Hoyos A : Relaciones Serologicas des los principales actinomycetes patogenes. Revta Inst. Salubr Enfern Trop Mex 13, 177-187, 1953.

105. Gonzales-Ochoa A and Baranda F : Unaprueba cutanea para el diagnostico del micetoma actinomicosico por Nocardia brasiliensis. Revt Inst Salubr Enferm Trop Mex 13, 189-197, 1953.

106. Gonzalez-Ochoa A and Sandoval DLC : Aislamiento de Nocardia brasiliensis and asteroides a partir de suelos. Revta Inst Salubr Enferm Trop Mex, 20, 147-151, 1960.

107. Gonzalez-Ochoa A : Mycetoma caused by Nocardia brasiliensis with a note on the the isolation of causative organism from soil. Lab 11, 1118-1123, 1962.

108. Gonzalez-Ochoa A. : Systemic mycoses. A CIBA foundation symposium in commemoration of WB Bikie, Edited by Wolstenholme and Porter. J & A Churchill Ltd. London, 1968.

109. Gonzalez-Ochoa A : Virulence of Nocardiae. Cand J Microbiol 19, 901, 1973.

110. Gonzalez-Ochoa A and Sandoval-Vuellar A : Different degree of morbidity in the white mouse induced by Nocardia brasiliensis. N. asteroides and N.caviae. Sabouraudia, 14, 255-259, 1976.

111. Gordon RE and Smith MM : Proposed group of characters for the separation of Streptomyces and Nocardia. J. Bact 69, 147-150, 1955.

112. Gordon RE and Mihm JM : The type species of genus Nocardia. J. Gen Microbiol 27, 1-10, 1962.

113. Green WO and Adams TE : Mycetoma in United states - A review and report of seven additional cases. Am J Clin Path. 42, 75-91, 1964.

114. Grueber HLE and Kumar TM : Mycetoma caused by Streptomyces somaliensis in North India. Sabouraudia, 8, 108-111, 1970.

115. Gugnani HC, Suseelan AV, Ude FN and Ojukwu JD : Actinomycetoma in Nigeria. J Trop Med and Hyg. 84, 259, 1981.

116. Gugnani HC, Ojukwand JD et al . : Mycetoma of tumb caused by Nocardia transvalensis. 80, 35-40, 1983.

117. Gugnani HC, Unaogu IC : Experimental mycetoma due to Streptomyces griseus in the laboratory mice. Mycopathologia 113(3), 151-154, 1991.

118. Gupta SK, Shukla VK and Khanna S : Primary actinomycotic mycetoma of anterior abdominal wall (A case report). J Post Grad Med 36(3), 175-177, 1990.

119. Hassan AM and Mahgoub ES : Lymphnode involvement in mycetoma. Trans Royal Soc Trop Med and Hyg 66, 165, 1972.

120. Hay RJ and Collins MJ : An ultrastructural study of pale eumycetoma grains. Sabouraudia, 21, 261-269, 1983.

121. Hay RJ, Mackenzie DWR : Mycetoma (Madura foot) in the United Kingdom - A study of 44 cases. Clin Exp Dermatol 8, 553-562, 1983.

122. Hemashettar BM, Patil CS, Nagalotimath S and Thammayya A : Mycetoma due to Exophiala jeanselmei (A case report with description of fungus). Indian J Pathol Microbiol 29, 75-78, 1986.

123. Huerre M, Ravisse P, Dubourdieu D, Morillon M, McCarthy S, Bobin S : Deep mycoses observed in New Caledonia. Evaluation of observations from laboratory of pathologic anatomy of the Pasteur Institute of New Caledonia 1975-1990. Bull Soc Pathol Exot 84(3) 247-256, 1991.

124. Indira PU and Sirsi M: tudies on maduromycosis. Indian J. Med. Res. 56, 1265-1271, 1968.

125. Jameson JE : Rapid and sensitive precipitin test for the diagnosis of farmer's lung using immuno-osmophoresis. J Clin Path 21, 376-382, 1968.

126. Jeanselme L, Huel E and Lotte F : Nouvean type de mycetoma a grains noirs due a Uno Torula non encore decrite. Soc Ft Dermatol Syph 5, 369, 1928.

127. Joshi KR, Sran HS, Ramdeo IN et al. : Clinicomycologic study of mycetoma - Proceedings 21st Annual meeting of Indian Association of Pathologist Pondicherri 1971.

128. Joshi KR, Sran HS, Ramdeo IN and Sachdev KN : Mycetoma caused by Madurella grisea in India. Indian J Derm and Venereol 39(1), 1-4, 1973.

129. Joshi KR, Mathur DR, Sharma K and Chawala SN : Mycetoma caused by Streptomyces pelletieri. Indian J Dermatol Venereol Lepr 46(2), 123-125, 1980.

130. Joshi KR, Mathur DR, Sharma JC, Vyas MCR and Sanghvi A : Mycetoma caused by Aspergillus nidulans in India. J Trop Med Hyg. 88, 41-44, 1985.

131. Joshi KR, Sanghvi A, Vyas MCR and Sharma JC : Etiology and distribution of mycetoma in Rajasthan. Indian J Med Res, 85, 694-698, 1987.

132. Joshi KR and Singhvi S. : Serodiagnosis of mycetoma. Trans Royal Soc Trop Med Hyg 82, 334, 1988.

133. Kakoty LM and Dey NC : Mycetoma caused by Glenospora semoni. Indian J Med Sci 11, 889, 1956.

134. Klokke AH : Mycetoma in North India due to Nocardia brasiliensis. Trop Geogr Med 162, 170-171, 1964.

135. Klokke AH : Abstract of the paper from report on IIIrd symposium. Dermatologicum Internationale Sub auspiciis societatis. Internationalis Dermatologiae Tropicale Brastislava. Mycopath Mycol Appl 31, 341, 1967.

136. Klokke AH, Swami DG, Angul R, Verghese A : The causal agents of mycetoma in South India. Trans Royal Soc Trop Med Hyg 62, 509-516, 1968.

137. Koshi G, Victor N and Chacko J : Causal agents in mycetoma of foot in south India. Sabouraudia 10, 14, 1972.

138. Koshi G, Kurian T, Mathai R, Abraham J, Joseph LBM and Selvapandian AJ. : Diverse etiologic agents from mycetoma cases. Indian J Med Res 74, 539-543, 1981.

139. Krassik SL, Subramanyam L, Green R and Book J. : Disseminated Nocardia brasiliensis infection. Archieves Dermatol, 112, 370, 1976.

140. Kulowaski J and Stovall J. : Maduromycosis of tibia in native Americans. J Amer Med Assoc 135, 429-432, 1947.

141. Kumar R and Mohapatra LN : Studies in aerobic actiomycetes - Isolation and identification of strain. Sabouraudia 6, 140, 1968.

142. Kurup PV, Randhawa HS, Sandhu RS and Abraham : Pathogenicity of Nocardia caviae. N. asteroides and N.brasiliensis. Mycopatho Mycol Appl 40, 113, 1970.

143. Langeron M : Mycetoma-Torula jeanselmei Nouveau type de mycetoma a grains noirs. Ann Parasitol Hum Com, 6, 385, 1928.

144. Latapi F : Griseofulvin in the treatment of some deep mycoses. Arch Derm, 81, 841-848, 1960.

145. Latapi F and Ortiz Y : Los micetoma en Mexico, Algunos Datos Nuevos Clinilos and Epidemiologicus Relatives A 197 cases. Memorias del Primer Congreso Mexicano de dermatologia. Mexico DF, 1, 126-144, 1963.

146. Lavalle P : Clinica Y Terapeutica de los micetoma. Derm Int 5, 117-120, 1966.

147. Lechevalier HA and Lechevalier MP : A critical evaluation of the genera of Aerobic actinomycetes In Prauser H ed. The Actinomycetales. Jena; Gustav Fischer Verlag, 1970.

148. Leslie C, Albert B and Max S : Pathogenesis of mycetoma. In Topley ad Wilson Microbiology and Microbial Infection, 9th ed. Vol - 4 Medical Mycology, volume editors Libero A and Roderick JH. Arnold Publication, pg 489, 1998.

149. Lewall DB, Ofole S and Bendle BJ : Mycetoma Skeletal Radiology, 14, 257, 1985.

150. L Opez Mart inez R, Mendez Tovar LJ, Lavelle P, Welsh O, Saul A, Macotel Runiz E : Epidemiology of mycetoma in Mexico-Study of 2105 cases. Gac Med Mex 128, 477-481, 1992.

151. Ludwin EH and Hutchinson WG : A serological study of selected species of Actinomyces. J Bact 58, 141-151, 1949.

152. Lynch JB : Mycetoma in Sudan. Ann R Coll Surg 35, 319-340, 1964.

153.Machado LA, Rivitfi Mc, Cuce LC, Salebian A, Lacaz C da S, Heins Vaccari EM, Belda Junior W, de Malo NT : Black grain eumycetma due to Madurella grisea - A report of 2 cases. Rev Inst Med Trop Sao Paulo 34(6), 569-80, 1992.

154.Mackinnon JE, Ferrada LV and Montemayor L : Investigaciones sobre las maduromicosis Y sus agents. An Fac Med Univ Montevideo, 34, 231-300, 1949(a).

155.Mackinnon JE, Ferrada LV and Montemayor L : Madurella grisea N. Sp. - A new species of fungus producing the black variety of maduromycosis in South America. Mycopath Mycol Appl 4, 385-392, 1949(b).

156.Mackinnon JE : Characteristicas de cuatro cultivos de Madurella mycetomi (Laveran) Brumpt aislados en el sudan y en la Somalia Britannica. An Fac Med Univ Montevideo, 36, 197-210, 1951.

157.Mackinnon JE : A contribution to the study of causal organisms of maduromycosis. Trans R Soc Trop Med Hyg 48, 470-480, 1954.

158.Mackinnon JE and Vidal S. : Caracteres differenciales entre la form a parasitaria de Madurella mycetomi y la de Madurella grisea. Arches Soc Biol Montevideo 21, 36-43, 1954.

159.Mackinnon JE and Artagaveytia - Allende RC : The main species of pathogenic aerobic actinomycetes causing mycetoma. Trans R Soc. Trop Med Hyg 51, 31-40, 1956.

160.Mackinnon JE, Artagaveytia - Allende RC and Garcia - Zooron N. : The inhibitary effect of chemotherapeutic agents on the growth of the causal organisms of exogenous mycetomas and Nocardias. Trans R Soc Trop Med Hyg 52, 78-86, 1958.

161.Magnusson M : Specificity of sensitins, further studies on guinea pigs with sensitins of various species of Mycobacteria and Nocardia. Am Rev Res Dis, 86, 395-404, 1962.

162.Mahgoub ES : The value of gel diffusion in diagnosis of mycetoma. Trans R Soc Trop Med Hyg 58, 560-563, 1964.

163.Mahgoub ES : Mycotic infections in Sudan Thesis for PhD University of London, 1965.

164.Mahgoub ES: Clinical aspects of Mycetoma systemic mycoses. A CIBA Foundation Symposium J & A Churchill Ltd. London. Pp 125-127 1968.

165.Mahgoub ES : Maduromycetoma caused by Aspergillus nidulans. J Trop Med Hyg 74, 60-61, 1971.

166.Mahgoub ES : Treatment of actinomycetoma with sulfamethoxazole and trimethoprim. Am J Trop Med and Hyg 21, 332-333, 1972.

167.Mahgoub ES and Murray IG : Mycetoma. William Heinemann Medical Book Ltd. London 1973.

168.Mahgoub ES : Medical Management of mycetoma. World Health Organisation 54, 303-309, 1976.

169.Mahgoub ES, Gumma SA, El Hassan AM : Immunological status of mycetoma patients Bull Soc Pathol Exot 70, 48-54, 1978.

170.Mahgoub ES and Gumma SA : Ketaconazole in the treatment of eumycetoma due to Madurella mycetomi. Trans R Soc Trop Med Hyg 78, 376-379, 1984.

171.Maiti PK and Halder PK : Mycetoma in exposed and non-exposed parts of body. A study of 212 cases. Indian J Med Microbiol 16(1), 19-22, 1998.

172.Malik AK, Sabharwal U, Chugh TD : Isolation characterisation and animal pathogenicity of Nocardia isolated from soil. Indian J Pathol Microbiol 25, 263-267, 1982.

173.Mankodi RC and Kanvindo MS : Mycetoma - A histological study. J Indian Med Assoc 54, 405, 1970.

174.Mariat F and Satre J : Action de la sulphamethoxypyridazine sur queiques actinomycetes aerobies pathogenes. Bull Soc Path Exot 54, 63-70, 1961.

175.Mariat F : Surla distribution geographique et la repartition des agents des mycetomes. Bull Soc Path Exot 56, 35-45, 1963.

176.Mathur DR, Joshi KR and Mathur A. : An aetiological and pathological study of mycetoma in Western Rajasthan. Curr Med Pract 23, 151-160, 1979.

177.Mathur DR, Agarwal SC : Mycetoma in Nigeria - A review. Nigerian Med Pract. II (3), 79-81, 1986.

178.Mathur DR, Bhardwaj V, Vaishnav K and Ramdeo IN : Red grain mycetoma caused by Actinomadurae pelletieri in Western Rajasthan. Report of two cases. Indian J Pathol Microbiol, 36(4), 486-488, 1993.

179. Mathur DR, Prakash P, Gupta PC, Purohit A, Vyas MCR : Red grain mycetoma in Western Rajasthan Indian. J Dermatol Venerol Leprol 60, 99-100, 1994.

180. Maya S and Basu N. : Aetiology of mycetoma cases. Bull Cal Sch Trop Med Hyg 2, 115, 1964.

181. Mc Elory JA. De Almeida Prestecs C. Su WP: Mycotoma infection with tumification, draining sinuses and grains. Cutis. 49(2_

182. Mc Ginnis MR and Padhye AA : Exophiala jeanselmei a new classification for Phialophora jeanselmei, Mycotaxon 5, 341, 1977.

183. McGinnis MR, D'Amato RF and Land GA : Differentiation of selected aerobic actinomycetes, In Pictorial hand book of medically important fungi and other aerobic actinomycetes. Praeger Publishers, NewYork, 1982.

184. Mirza SH and Campbell C : Mycetoma caused by Nocardia transvalensis. J Clin Pathol, 47(1), 85-86, 1994.

185. Mishra SK and Randhawa HS. : Observations on paraffin baiting as a laboratory diagnostic procedure in nocardiosis Mycopath Mycol Appl 51, 147, 1973.

186. Mishra SK, Sandhu RS, Randhawa VN, Damodaran and Abraham: Effect of cortisone administration on experimental Nocarsiosis. Infec and Immunity 7, 123-129, 1973.

187. Mishra SK, Gordon RE and Barnet A : Identification of Nocardiae and Streptomyces of medical importance. J Clin Microbiol 11, 728-736, 1980.

188. Moghraby IM : Mycetoma in the Gezira a public health problem. Commun vi Arab Med Conf (Khartoum) 1967.

189. Mohanty PK, Ambedkar VA, Deodhar LP, Ranada R, Mehta VR : Nocardia brasiliensis - mycetoma. J Postgrad Med 28, 179-180, 1982.

190. Mohapatra LN and Pine L : Studies on the pathogenicity of aerobic actinomycetes inoculated into mice intravenously. Sabouraudia. 2, 176, 1963.

191. Mohapatra LN and Bhargava S : Mycetoma Indian J Ortho 1, 173, 1967.

192. Murray IG, Spooner ETC and Walker J : Experimental infection of mice with Madurella mycetomi. Trans R Soc Trop Med Hyg 54, 335-341, 1960.

193.Murray IG: Report to the Medical Research Council on visit to Sudan. 1960.

194.Murray IG and Colichon H : Chemotherapy of maduromycosis. Trans R Soc. Trop Med Hyg 56, 156-165, 1962.

195.Murray IG and Holt HD : Is Cephalosporium acremonium capable of producing maduromycosis ? Mycopath Mycol Appl 22, 335-338, 1964.

196.Murray IG and Moghraby IM : The value of skin test in distinguishing between maduromycetoma and actinomycetoma. Trans R Soc Trop Med Hyg 58, 557-559, 1964.

197.Murray IG and Mahgoub ES : Further studies in the diagnosis of mycetoma by double diffusion in agar. Sabouraudia,6, 106-110, 1968.

198.Murti BR and Padmavati DC : Study of aetiology of mycetoma. Indian J Microbiol 3, 99-103, 1963.

199.Nasher M, Wethered DB et al. : An ultrastructural study of Streptomyces somaliensis grains in vivo and vitro. Am J Hyg Trop Med 37, 174-179, 1987.

200.Nauhauser I : Black grain maduromycosis caused by Madurella grisea. Arch Derm 72, 351-352, 1955.

201.Nelson E and Henrici AI : Immunological studies of Actinomycetes with special reference to the acid fast species. Proc Soc Exp Biol Med 19, 351-352, 1922.

202.Neurmeister W, Zolliner TM, Krieger D, Sterry W., Marre R : Mycetoma due to Exophiala jeanselmei and Mycobacterium chelonae in a 73 year old man with idiopathic CD4+ T lymphopenia. Mycoses, 38(7-8), 271-276, 1995.

203.Nicholle C and Pinoy E : Sur Un cas de mycetome d'origine aspergillaire observe en tunise Achieve de Parasitologic Paris, 10, 437-438, 1906.

204.Nityananda K : Mycotic diseases in Ceylon. Ceylon Med J, 1, 197-207, 1962.

205.Orio J, Destombes P, Mariat F and Segretain G : Les Mycetomes en cote Francaise des Somalis. Revue de 50 cas observes enter 1954 et 1962. Bull Soc Path Exot 56, 161-173, 1963.

206.Oyston JK : Madura foot, a study of twenty cases. J Bone Joint-Surg (Brit) 43B, 259-267, 1961.

207.Pankajlaxmi VV and Taralaxmi : Small grain mycetomas in the tropics. Aust J Dermatol, 23, 39-42, 1982.

208.Pankajlaxmi VV and Taralaxmi VV : Mycetoma in Tropics. Indian J Pathol Microbiol 27, 223-228, 1984.

209.Pankajlaxmi VV and Taralaxmi VV : Red grain mycetoma of scalp due to Actinomadura pelletieri in Madurai. Indian J Pathol Microbiol 33, 384-86, 1990.

210.Panja G and Chaudhari SN : Mycetoma foot of melanoid variety. Indian J Derm and Venerol 3, 24, 1958.

211.Peerapur BV and Inamadar AC : Mycetoma of scalp due to Nocardia brasiliensis. Indian J Pathol Microbiol 15, 85-86, 1997.

212.Philippon M, Larroque D, Ravisse P : Mycetoma in Mauritania - Species found epidemiologic characters and country distribution. Report of 122 cases. Bull Soc Pathol Exot, 85(2), 107-174, 1992.

213.Pinoy E : Actinomycoses et mycetoma. Bull Inst Pasteur, 11, 929-938, 977-984, 1913.

214.Prats E, Sans J, Valldeperas J, Ferrer JE, Manresa E : Pulmonary mycetoma like lesion caused by Candida tropicalis. Respir Med 89(4) 303-304, 1995.

215.Proctor AGJ : Pathogenic Streptomyces. J Med Lab Technol 23, 109-114, 1966.

216.Rajendran C and Kandhari S : Mycetoma due to Nocardia brasiliensis. First case report from the union territory of Delhi. Mycoses, 32(9), 476-481, 1989.

217.Rajendran C, Baby A, Kumari S, Verghese T. An evaluation of straw-extract agar media for the growth and sporulation of Madurella mycetomatis. Mycopathologia, 115, 9-12, 1991.

218.Reddy CRRM, Sundareshwar B, Pattabhirama RA, Reddy SS : Mycetoma-Histological diagnosis of causal agents in 50 cases of mycetoma. Indian J Med Sci 26, 733-736, 1972.

219.Reifferschied M and Seeliger H : Monosporiose und Maduromycose. Dt Med Wschr 80, 1841, 1955.

220.Rey M : Les mycetomes dans l'quest - Africain Theese R Foulon and Company Paris, 1961.

221.Reyes AC : A contribution to the study of mycetoma in Philippines Maduromycosis caused by Monosporium apiospermum (laboratory studies). 19, 89-102, 1963.

222.Sakand eB, Traor sS, Kabor eJ, Quattara T, Soudr eRB : Human parasitoses in Burikino Faso Histopathologic approach. Bull Soc Pathol Exot 91(3), 217-220, 1998.

223.Salinas Carmona MC, Vera L, Welsch O, Rodriguiz M. Antibody response to Nocardia brasiliensis antigens in man. Int J Med Microbiol Virol Parasitol Infect Dis. 276(3), 390-397, 1992.

224.Salinas-Carmona MC, Welsh O and Casillas SM. : Enzyme-linked immunosorbent assay for serological diagnosis of Nocardia brasiliensis and clinical correlation with mycetoma. J Clin Microbiol, 33(11), 2901-2906, 1993.

225.Salinas-Carmona MC and Torres-L Opez E : Role of passive humoral immunity in experimental mycetoma by Nocardia brasiliensis. Ann NY Acad Sci 797, 263-265, 1996.

226.Salinas-Carmona MC, Castro-Corno MA, Sepulveda-Saavedra J and Perez LJ : Monoclonal antibodies to P24 and P61 immunodominant antigens from Nocardia brasiliensis. Clin Diagn Lab Immunol, 4(2), 133-137, 1997.

227.Sankhala SS, Sharma JC, Vyas MCR, Mehta MC : Mycetoma of the same foot caused by Madurella mycetomi and Streptomyces somaliensis - A case report. Indian J Orth 21(1), 94-96, 1987.

228.Sanyal M and Basu N : On the aetiology of mycetoma cases. Bull Cal Sch Trop Med, 12, 115-118, 1964.

229.Saraca GD, Towersey L, Bay RJ, Londero AT, Mortins E de, Amora AT, Reis KM, Mendonca AM : Mycetoma by Nocardia asteroides a nine year followup. Rev Inst Med Trop Sao Paulo 35(2), 199-204, 1993.

230.Schmitt JA, Zabransky RJ, Janidlo AS and Parson JE : Experimental maduromycosis in the laboratory mouse. Mycopath Mycol Appl 18, 164-168, 1962.

231.Schneidau JA and Shaffer MF : Studies on Nocardia and other Actinomycetes, antigenic relationship shown by slide agglutination tests. Am Rev Res Dis, 82, 64-76, 1960.

232. Sebastiao AP, Sampaio C and Silva L : Acao do sulfisoxazol na actinomycose provocada pelo A.brasiliensis. Hospital Rio De J, 50, 795-802, 1956.

233. Segretain G : Sur les phialides et phialospores produites par Madurella mycetomi. Cir Scan Acad Sci 247, 130-132, 1958.

234. Segretain G, Destombes P. : Description d'um nouvel agent de maduromycoses, Neotestudina rosatii, n sp isole en Afrique. CR Acad SCi Paris, 253, 2577-2579, 1961.

235. Segretain G : Some new or infrequent fungus pathogens. In Fungi and Fungal diseases, Dulldorf G ed, Springfield, Charles C Thomas, pg 33-49, 1962.

236. Segretain G and Destombes P : Les mycetomes en Afrique du Nord. Maroc Med 42, 445-450, 1963.

237. Segretain G, Mariat F : Recherches sur la presence d'agents de mycetomes dans le sol et sur les epineux du Senegal et de la Mauritanie. Bull Soc Pathol Exot 62, 194-202, 1969.

238. Segretain G, Andre M, Sarrat HET, Destombes P : Leptosphaeria tompkinsii, agent de mycetomes an Senegal. Bull Soc Fr Mycol Med 3, 71-74, 1974.

239. Sharif HS, Clark DC, Aabed MY, Aideyan OA, Mattsson TA, Haddad MC, Joshi RK, Hasan HA, Haleem A : Mycetoma comparison of MR imaging with CT. Radiology 178(3), 865-870, 1991.

240. Sharma JC, Joshi KR, Vyas MCR, Sankhala SS, Gupta SP : Mycetoma caused by Streptomyces somaliensis in Jodhpur (India). Indian J Med Microbiol, 5, 213-221, 1987.

241. Sharma JC, Joshi KR, Vyas MCR, Sankhala SS and Gupta SP. A clinicopathological and mycological study of mycetoma involving upper extrimity at Jodhpur, India. Indian J Med Sci, 42(5) 103-108, 1988.

242. Sharma JC, Joshi KR, Vyas MCR, Sankhala SS and Gupta SP. Mycetoma in Jodhpur division of Western Rajasthan. Indian J Orth 24, 18-26, 1990.

243. Shelly MA, Poe RH, Kapner LB : Pulmonary mycetoma due to Candida albicans, case report and review. Clin Infect Dis, 22(1), 133-135, 1996.

244. Siano VI, Budumian TM and Piankova OM : Mycetoma of Hand. Vestn Dermatol Venerol 11, 56-59, 1990.

245.Silva M do R, Fernandes D de F, Oliveira LM, Costa MB and Castro LC : Madurella grisea eumycetoma, presentation of a case. Rev Soc Bras Med Trop, 24(1), 51-54, 1991.

246.Singh H : Black grain perinal mycetoma. Indian J Surg. 38(12), 530-534, 1976.

247.Singh H : Mycetoma in India. Indian J. Surg. 41(10), 577-597, 1979.

248.Singh H : Mycetoma-clinical staging, classification and management. Presented at 1st National Symposium on Mycetoma : 26-28th Feb. 1998 at Dr. S.N. Medical College Jodhpur Rajasthan India.

249.Singh M and Sandhu RS : Environmental prevalence of Nocardia species in Punjab state (India). Indian J Med Res 82, 402-407, 1985.

250.Singhvi AM, Singh SP, Malviya S, Makwana S : Extrapedal mycetoma - A study of 108 cases. SDMH J 19(3), 113-117, 1995.

251.Singhvi AM, Malviya A, Joshi KR : A study of prevalence of mycetoma fungi in Jodhpur region. ICMR Project, 1995a.

252.Singhvi A, Joshi KR, Sharma JC and Vyas MCR : Immunoglobulin profile in mycetoma. Indian J Pathol Microbiol 39, 203-206, 1996.

253.Southern PM Jr. : Mycetoma due to Madurella grisea acquired in Mexico. Trop Doct 26(4), 187-188, 1996.

254.Sran HS and Joshi KR : Mycetoma of upper extrimity. Jap J Surg 2(2), 86-91, 1972.

255.Sran HS, Bothra VC, Narula IMS, Joshi KR and Agarwal GR : Clinical study of mycetoma. Indian J Dermatol and Venerol, 39(3), 141-148, 1973.

256.Subrahamanyam M : Intra-arterial chemotherapy for mycetoma of foot. Br. J Surg 82(5), 643, 1995.

257.Suttner JF, Wirth CJ, Wulker N, Seeliger H : Madura foot. Int Orthop, 14, 217-219, 1990.

258.Talwar P and Sehgal SC : Mycetoma in North India. Sabouraudia, 17, 287-291, 1979.

259.Tambaku SN and Sengupta SR : Mycetoma foot A report of six cases. Indian J Surg 31, 56-61, 1969.

260.Thammayya A and Sanyal M : Expophiala jeanselmei causing mycetoma pedis in India, Sabouraudia 18, 91, 1980.

261. Turiansky GM, Benson PM, Sperling LC, Sau P, Salkin IF, McGinnis MR, James WD : Phialophora verrucosa - A new cause of mycetoma. J Am Acad Dermatol 32, 311-315, 1995.

262. Uppal MS, Kohman LJ and Katzenstein AL : Mycetoma with in an intralobar sequestration, evidence supporting acquired origin for this pulmonary anomaly. Chest 103(5), 1627-1628, 1993.

263. Unaogu IC, Gugnani HC and Ikerionwu SE : Experimental actinomycetoma due to Nocardia transvalensis in laboratory mice. Mycoses 33(2), 99-102, 1990.

264. Unaogu IC and Gugnani HC : Pathogenicity of Streptomyces griseus for laboratory mice. Mycoses 33(3), 146-150, 1990.

265. Vanbreuseghem R and Bernaerts JP : Production experimental de grains maduromycosiques par Monosporium apiospermum et Allescheria boydii. Annls Soc Belge Med Trop, 35, 451-456, 1955.

266. Vanbreuseghem R : Epidemiologic et therapeutique de pieds de madura au Congo Belge. Bull Soc Pathol Exot, 51,793-814, 1958.

267. Venbreuseghem R : Early diagnosis treatment and epidemiology of mycetoma. Rev Med Vet Mycol 6, 49, 1967.

268. Verghese A and Klokke AH : Histologic diagnosis of species causing mycetoma. Indian J Med Res 54, 524, 1966.

269. Verghese SL, Madhavan HN and Sekar B : Isolation and characterisation of Nocardia from clinical specimen. J Indian Med Assoc 94(2), 58-59, 1996.

270. Venugopal TV and Venugopal PV : Mycetoma in Madras. Sabouraudia, 15, 17-22, 1977.

271. Venugopal PV, Venugopal TV, Laing WM, al Humaidan Y, Namnyak SS, al Jama AA, Elbashier AM : Black grain mycetoma caused by Madurella grisea in Saudi Arabia. Int J Dermatol 29(6), 434-435, 1990.

272. Venugopal PV and Venugopal TV : Red grain mycetoma of scalp due to Actinomadura pelletieri in Madurai Indian J Pathol Microbiol, 33(4), 384-386, 1990a.

273. Venugopal PV and Venugopal TV : Leptosphaeria tompkinsii in mycetoma. Int J Dermatol 29(6), 432-433, 1990b.

274. Venugopal PV and Venugopal TV : Actinomadura madurae causing mycetomas in Madras. Indian J Pathol Microbiol 34(2), 119-125, 1991.

275. Venugopal PV and Venugopal TV : Treatment of eumycetoma with Ketoconazole. Australas J Dermatol 34(1), 27-29, 1993.

276. Venugopal PV and Venugopal TV : Antimycotic susceptibility testing of agents of black grain eumycetoma. J Med Vet Mycol 31(2) 161-164, 1993a.

277. Venugopal PV and Venugopal TV : Pale grain eumycetoma in Madras. Australas J Dermatol 36(3), 149-151, 1995.

278. Vincent MH : Etude sur le parasite du pied de madura. Annls Inst Pasteur Paris 8, 129-151, 1894.

279. Walker RM, Ashdown IR, Magurie EJ : Beneficial effects of hyperbaric oxygen therapy in Nocardia brasiliensis soft tissue infection. Med J Aust. 155(2), 122-123, 1991.

280. Wanke NC, Wanke B, Caiuby MJ, Towersay L, Londero AT, Dias MF, Siqueira SP : Mycetoma due to Actinomadura madurae A report of 2 cases. Rev Inst Med Trop Sao Paulo 34(4) 367-372, 1992.

281. Welsch O, Sauceda E, Gonzalez J, Ocampo J : Amikasin alone and in combination with trimethoprim-sulfamethoxazole in the treatment of actinomycotic mycetoma. J Am Acad Dermatol 17, 443-448, 1987.

282. Welsch O, Salinas MC, Rodriquez MA : Treatment of eumycetoma and actinomycetoma. Curr Trop Med Mycol, 6, 47-71, 1995.

283. Wethered DB, Markey MA et al. Ultrastructure and immunogenic changes in the formation of mycetoma grain. J Med Vet Mycol 25, 39-46, 1987.

284. Wethered DB, Markey MA et al. : Humoral immune response to mycetoma organisms, characterisation of specific antibodies by use of enzyme linked immunosorbent assay and immunoblotting. Trans R Soc Trop Med Hyg 82, 918-923, 1988.

285. Wilson AMM : The aetiology of mycetoma in Uganda compared with other African Countries. E Afr Med J 42, 182-190, 1965.

286. Winslow DT and Steen: Consideration in the histologic diagnosis of mycetoma. Am J Clin Path 42, 164-169, 1964.

287. Witzig RS, Greer DL, Hyslop NE Jr : Aspergillus flavus mycetoma and epidural abscess successfully treated with itraconazole. J Med Vet Mycol 34(2) 133-137, 1996.

288. Wortman PD : Treatment of Nocardia brasiliensis in mycetoma with sulfamethoxazole and trimethoprim, amikacin and amoxicillin and clavulanate. Arch Dermatol 129(5), 564-567, 1993.

289. Young BB and Hotchkiss M : Developmental morphology in the genus Nocardia. Mycopath. Mycol Appl, 11, 297-310, 1959.

290. Yu AM, Zhao S, Nie LY : Mycetomas in Northern Yemen - Identification of causative organisms and epidemiological considerations. Am J Trop Med Hyg 48(6), 812-817, 1993.

291. Zaias N and Taplin D : Mycetoma. Arch Dermatol 99, 215-225, 1969.

292. Zamora A, Bojalil LF and Bastarrachea F : Immunologically active polysaccharide from Nocardia asteroids and Nocardia brasiliensis. J Bact 85, 549-555, 1962.

293. Ziprowsky L, Altmann G, Dalith F and Spitz V : Mycetoma pedis four cases treated with streptomycin. Arch Derm. 75, 855-863, 1957.

294. Zoutman DE and Sigler L : Mycetoma of foot caused by Clinodrocarpon destructans. J. Clin Microbiol 29(9), 1855-1859, 1991.

Appendix

Isolation and Identification of Etiological Agents of Mycetoma

INTRODUCTION

Mycetoma is a granulomatous infection characterized by subcutaneous tumefactions or swellings, usually on the lower limbs with sinuses that generally discharge pus containing granules of varying colour. Two main types of mycetoma are recognized, namely actinomycetoma caused by actinomycetes and eumycetoma caused by true fungi. The principal etiological agents of actinomycetoma are *Nocardia brasiliensis*, *N. otitidiscaviarum*, *Actinomadura madurae*, *A. pelletieri*, *N. asteroides*, *Nocardiopsis dassonvillei*, *Streptomyces somaliensis* (Dasgupta et al, 1974; Sandhu et al, 1975; Sanyal et al 1978; Gugnani et al, 1981; Pankajlakshmi & Taralakshmi, 1984; Joshi et al, 1987; Rippon, 1988; Kwon-Chung & Bennett, 1992; McNeil & Brown, 1994; Verghese & Klokke, 1996). *Nocardia transvalensis*, *S. albus* and *S. griseus* are occasional agents of actinomycetoma (Gugnani et al, 1982; McNeil &Brown, 1994); however they have not been so far reported from India. The main fungal etiological agents of mycetoma include *Madurella mycetomatis*, *M. grisea*, *Pseudallescheria boydii*, *Leptosphaeria senegalensis*, *Exophiala jeanselmei*, *Neotestudina rosatii*, *Pyrenochaeta romeroi*, *Acremonium kiliense*, *A. falciforme* and *A. recifei* (Kandhari et al, 1964; Indira & Sirsi, 1965; Mahgoub & Murray, 1973; Thammaya & Sanyal 1973, 1980; Joshi et al,

1987; Koshi et al, 1972, 1979; Pankajlakshmi & Taralakshmi, 1984; Rippon, 1988; Kwon-Chung & Bennett, 1992; Verghese & Klokke, 1996)

DEMONSTRATION OF ETIOLOGICAL AGENTS IN GRANULES AND THEIR ISOLATION IN CULTURE

The pus discharged from sinuses is collected and is examined for granules (grains) which are aggregates of actinomycotic or fungal filaments. The granules are basic material for identification and culture. In the absence of discharging granules, a deep wedge-shaped biopsy is taken around a sinus. Half of the specimen is sent for histopathology in 10 % formal saline and the other half is dissected under a x 4 lens or a dissecting microscope and grains are picked out. The grains are rinsed in sterile normal saline and crushed. Portions of the crushed granules are examined in 10% or 20% KOH mounts for presence of true fungal hyphae and associated structures. Smears of the material of crushed granules are stained by Gram and Kinyoun`s acid fast stain and examined for presence of thin Gram positive actinomycotic hyphae that may be acid-fast. The remaining portions of the crushed granules are cultured on appropriate media, viz. glucose (1%) nutrient agar, blood agar and McClung`s broth with paraffin coated rods suspended therein, in case an aerobic actinomycete is suspected as the etiological agent. If a true fungus is suspected as the etiological agent, the material is cultured on Sabouraud`s agar, brain heart infusion agar and blood agar supplemented with chloramphenicol (0.05 mg/ml) alone or with chloramphenicol and cycloheximide (0.5 mg/ml). Slopes of agar media are better than plates for culturing clinical specimens. Cultures are incubated in half sets at 25 ^{0}C and 37 ^{0}C and regularly examined for suggestive growth for up to three weeks and purified by sub-culturing.

SPECIES IDENTIFICATION OF ACTINOMYCETES CAUSING MYCETOMA

Histological identification of the etiological agent is often possible by a detailed study of the grain (granules) in the tissue sections. Precise identification of pathogenic actinomycetes is done on the basis of colonial characters, microscopic features and biochemical characteristics. Gross colonial characteristics of the organism and production of the diffusible pigment are observed on 1% glucose nutrient agar for actinomycetes and on Sabouraud dextrose agar (SDA) for fungi. The gross characteristics of grains, their histological appearance and colonial and microscopic morphology of important pathogenic actinomycetes causing mycetoma are described in Table 1. The histological appearance of the grains of some of the etiological agents have been shown in chapter 8 of actinomycetoma. Colony characters often give a clue about the identity of the species. For instance, colonies of *Streptomyces somalienisis* are dirty yellow and turn black after 10 days. Colonies of *Actinomadura madurae* and *A. pelletieri* white and coral red respectively while that of *Nocardia brasiliensis* are biege or orange. Slide cultures on Sabouraud agar and tap water agar incubated at 30 ^{0}C to 35 ^{0}C for 7-10 days are examined to observe branching of filaments and spores. The colonial characters and microscopical features of some of the etiological agents of actinomycetoma are illustrated in chapter 9. Physiological tests for identification of actinomycetes include decomposition of amino acids and proteins along with the utilization of sugars. Appropriate positive and negative controls are included in each test series. Details of procedures for identification and preparation of required media and reagents have been described by Misra et al (1980), Land (1996) and Beneke & Rogers (1996). Briefly growth from one-week-old culture of a test isolate is streaked on one quadrant of a tyrosine plate, a xanthine and hypoxanthine plate. Plates are incubated for up to 2-3 weeks and zones of clearing of the crystals of the amino acids around the growth of the test isolate indicate decomposition of the respective amino acid. Casein hydrolysis is tested by inoculating on a medium containing skim milk (5%) and agar (2%). Plates are incubated for up to 2 weeks and examined for clearing of casein. Gelatin hydrolysis is tested by inoculating loopfuls of growth of the test isolates below the surface of nutrient broth gelatin tubes and incubating at the culture at 25 ^{0}C or 37 ^{0}C. After growth occurs, the tubes are refrigerated until control solidifies and checked for liquefaction. Nitrate reduction test is done as for bacteria. Lysozyme test is done by inoculating loopfuls of growth in a tube containing glycerol and lysozyme and incubated at room temperature for one week. Growth in lysozyme tube separates *Nocardia* species from *Streptomyces* and other aerobic actinomycetes. Urea hydrolysis is tested in Urea agar slopes or Urea broth. The salient differentiating biochemical features of aerobic actinomycetes causing mycetoma are given in Table 2. Several strains of aerobic acinomycetes, particularly those of *Nocardia* spp., *Actinomadura* spp. and *Streptomyces* spp. are variable in their morphological and physiological characteristics, posing difficulty in their generic identification. The chemical composition of cell wall of these strains is determined by thin layer chromatography or high-performance liquid chromatography. Whole-cell hydrolysates are used to detect the L-and meso-isomeres of diaminopimelic acid (DAP), the carbohydrate products (sugars) and the mycolic acid (Table 3.).

SPECIES IDENTIFICATION OF FUNGI CAUSING MYCETOMA

The gross and microscopic characteristics of grains are a useful aid in the identification of etiological agents of eumycetoma. The precise identification of fungi is based on observation of colonial morphology (consistency, colour, texture, rate of growth, topography, presence of diffusible or non-diffusible pigment on reverse) and microscopic features. Microscopic morphology, the major determinant for identification is best observed in slide cultures in SDA or Czapek-Dox agar. Sporulation is sometimes induced by inoculation on nutritionally deficient media such as cornmeal, carrot-potato, pea agar or on plain water agar. Physiological tests are in general of little value in identification, except for some species. The standard descriptions of the causal agents given by McGinnis (1980), Rippon (1988), Kwon-Chung & Bennett (1992) and Hoog & Guarro (1995) may be consulted. The gross and microscopic features of the grains in eumycetoma, and salient differentiating colonial and microscopic features of the etiological agents and distinguishing physiological characteristics of some of them are given in Table 4. The appearance of grains of most of the etiological agents of eumycetoma have been illustrated in chapter 9. The colonial and microscopical features of some of the etiological agents of eumycetoma are illustrated in chapter 9.

Table 1: Salient gross and histological features of grains, and colonial and microscopic features of pathogenic actinomycetes causing mycetoma (Adapted from Rippon, 1988; Kwon-Chung & Bennett, 1992; Verghese & Klokke, 1996)

Species	Grain morphology	Histology (H &E)	Colonial and Microscopic features
Nocardia brasilensis	White to yellow, lobular, soft, 0.5-1 mm	Homogenous, loose clumps of filaments with clubs	Glabrous, heaped, orange yellow or tan; branched mm filaments, rods, cocci, acid fast
N. otitidiscaviarum	White or yellow, lobular, <1.0 mm	Same as above	Glabrous, heaped, orange yellow; branched filaments, rods, cocci, acid-fast
N. asteroides	White yellow, soft Irregular, 1 mm	Same as above	Glabrous, folded, orange yellow; branched filaments, rods, cocci, acid-fast
*N. trans*valensis	Yellow, spherical, *lobed, 2 mm*	Homogenous, radiating *mass of filaments and* cocco-bacillary forms	Chalky white turning pink, *cerebreform, microscopic* morphology same as above
Actinomadura madurae	White to yellow oval, soft, 1 mm	Centre amorphous with dense basophilic periphery, wide pink border with loose fringe clubs	Cream white, occasionaly wrinkled glabrous; delicate, non fragmenting, branched, non acid-fast filaments
A. pelletieri	Red, hard, oval, or kidney-shaped hard, 0.3-0.5 mm	Periphery eosinophilic, centre stains intense with hematoxylene	Pink to red folded waxy; non-fragmenting filaments non acid-fast
Streptomyces somaliensis	Yellowish brown, spherical, hard, 0.5-2 mm	Amorphous, centre light purple with dark edge, breaking into fragments	Cream to brown wrinkled; substrate mycelium non-fragmenting; aerial mycelium non-acid fast, branched producing conidia in chains
Nocardiopsis dassonvillei	cream coloured, < 0.5 mm	Cream coloured, irregular, indistinguishable from those of *Nocardia* species	Yellow heaped up wrinkled colonies;. aerial hyphae long, branched appearing zigzag, later divide into long segments that subdivide into small elongate spores.

Table 2: Physiological characteristics of aerobic actinomycetes (Adapted from Kwin-Chung & Bennett, 1992; Land, 1996)

Species	Acid- Fast	L R.	Decomposition of:							Acid form:
			C	G	X	T	HX	U	N	
Nocardia asteroides	+	R	-	-	-	-	-	+	+	Gly
N. brasiliensis	+	R	+	+	-	+	+	+	+	Gly, Mn
N. otitidis caviarum	+	R	-	-	+	-	+	+	+	Gly, Arab
N. trans- valensis	+	R	-	-	-	+	+	+	+	Gly, Ery, Ml, Mn, Sorb
Actino- madura madurae	-	S	+	+	-	+	+	-	+	Gly, Arab, Cell, Xyl
A. pelletieri	-	S	+	+	-	+	+	-	+	Tre
Nocardiopsisdassonvillei	-	S	+	+	+	+	+	-	+	Gly, Cell Ml, Mn
Streptomyces somaliensis	-	S	+	+	-	+	-	-	V	Ml
S. albus	-	S	+	+	+	+	+	+	-	Cell, Gly Ery, La, MN Ml, Mb, Sorb
S. griseus	-	S	+	+	+	+	+	V	-	Gly, Lac, Ml Mn, Xyl

LR, Lysozyme Resistance; C, casein; G-gelatin; X, xanthine; T, tyrosine; HX, hypoxanthine; U, urea; N, nitrate reduction, +, positive; -, negative; V, variable ; * 15-80% of strains are positive. Gly-glycerol, Mn- mannose, Arab- arabinose, Ery-erythritol, Sorb-sorbitol, Tre- trehalose, Ml-mannitol, Cell-cellobiose, Mb-mellobiose, Lac-lactose, Xyl- xylose.

Table 3: Differentiation of genera of actinomycetes involved in actinomycetoma based on cell wall composition

Differentiating characteristic	*Actinomadura*	*Nocardia*	*Nocardioposis*	*Streptomyces*
Cell wall type	III/B; Meso-DAP, madurose	IV; Meso- DAP, arabinose, galactose	III/C; Meso-DAP no characteristic sugar	I; LL-DAP, glycine, no characteristic sugar
Nocardiomycolic acid	Absent	Present	Absent	Absent

DAP, Diaminopimelic acid

Table 4: Salient gross and histological features of grains, colonial and microscopical features, and physiological characteristics of fungi causing mycetoma

Species	Grain morphology	Histology (H &E)	Colonial, microscopic, Morphological and physiological features
Madurella mycetomatis	Black, hard, brittle oval to lobulated, < 2 mm, aggregated	Compact grains with dark cement between the light brown hyphae 1-5 μm wide containing brown particles, embedded in brown matrix; terminal swollen10-15 μm wide at the edge. Vesicular grains light brown with peripheral hyphae filled with vesicles6-15 μm wide	Moderately fast growing, yellow, olivaceous to brown frequently with brown diffusible pigment. Dense melanized mycelium with moniliform hyphae with large vesicle like cells; phialides with minute phialoconidida. sometimes produced on corn meal agar, sclerotia may be formed occasionally. Glucose galactose, lactose are utilized but not sucrose.
Madurella grisea	Black, soft, oval to lobulated < 1 mm polygonal cell at the periphery	Light coloured or non-pigmented central area	Very slow growing, tan gray, raised and folded, olivaceous to dark gray; sterile mycelim occasionally with chlamydo-conidia. Glucose, galactose, sucrose utilized but not lactose.

Species	Grain morphology	Histology (H &E)	Colonial, microscopic, Morphological and physiological features
Pyrenochaeta romeroi	Same as in *M. grisea*	Lacking cement with pale centre, periphery pigmented	Slow growing, velvety to floccose, gray to black, black with reverse olivace-ous black. Pycnidia black, submerged, subspherical; hyaline ellipsoid to elongate conidia ooze out in slimy drops. Pycnidia produced. only occasionally. Glucose, galactose, sucrose utilized but not lactose.
Pseudalle- scheria boydii(anamorph: *Scedosporium apiospermum*)	White or light yellow oval or lobulated, periphery pink > 1 mm	Hyaline hyphae 2-5 μm wide, centre with swollen globose to subglobose cells, 10-20 μm, periphery pink	Rapidly growing, fluffy mouse gray; unicellular, sub- spherical to elongate conidia on simple conidiophores. cleistothecia light brown to black with 8-spored asci evanescent; ascospores one 1-celled, lemon-shaped, pale yellow to golden brown with two terminal germ pores
Neotestudina rosatii	Soft, white or brown < 1 mm	Angulated mass breaking into sections containing filaments with polygonal cells, centre basophilic	Slow growing dark brown with radial grooves, reverse dark brown. Black, spherical cleistothecia with pseudo-parenchymatous peridium formed on corn meal or potato agar. Asci crescent to spherical, bitunicate, evanescent with eight2-celled brown, smooth thick walled ascospores
Leptosphaeria senegalensis	Black < 1.2 mm, tubular or hollow with dark periphery, comprised of dark hyphae with large vesicles	Centre contains light brown hyphae; periphery dark with brown cement and dark brown vesicles	Colonies slow growing, dark gray, floccose with reverse almost black. After4-8 weeks, black subspherical cleistothecia develop with brown thick walled peridium. Asci clavate, bitunicate, 8-spored; ascospores sub-hyaline, obovoidal to ellipsoidal, usually 4-septate constricted at septa with slimy

Species	Grain morphology	Histology (H &E)	Colonial, microscopic, Morphological and physiological features
			sheath.
Acremonium kiliense	White, soft, irregular, > 1.5 mm	Non-cemented, comprised of hyaline hyphae with swollen cells	Slow growing, ochracecous with reverse brown. Elliptical conidia produced in slimy balls at the tips of tapering phialides. Chlamydospores also seen.
Acremonium falciforme	White to pale yellow soft, < 1. 0 mm	No-cemented, comprised of dense mass of thin mycelium with swollen cells peripheral zone of radiating eosinophilic clubs	Slow growing, gray brown, becoming gray-violet with violet purple pigment on reverse; cylindrical to falcate1-3 celled conidia borne in mucoid clusters at the tips of undifferentiated conidiophores
Acremonium recifei	White to pale yellow, soft,< 1.5 mm	Non-cemented, comprised of brown dense mass of thin hylaine mycelium with swollen cells	Slow growing, white to pink ; reverse ochraceous brown; reinform conidia borne at the tips of tapering phialides, held together in ball in mucilaginous exudate, chlamydospores also seen
Exophiala jeanselmei	Black, soft, 0.2-0.3	Non-cemented, irregular to serpiginous, waxy, centre often hollow, comprised of brown hyphae with vesicular cells	Slow growing, black, moist turning velvety, reverse black, toruloid yeast cells. In old cultures, the hyphae form lagneifrom annelophores with ellipsoidal conidia borne in groups at the tips

ACKNOWLEDGEMENT

The author is very grateful to Dr. k. J. Kwon-Chung, Dr. M.D. Richardson, Dr. F.D. Chandler, Dr K. Safelder, Dr. A Thammaya and Dr Carlyn Halde, and the publishers: Lea & Febiger, Blackwell Science, Wolf Medical Publications Ltd., and Kluwer Academic Publishers for their kind permission to reproduce some of their illustrations in this Chapter

REFERENCES

1. Bennett ES & Rogers AL. (1996) Medical Mycology and Human Mycoses, pp 99-105, 215-219 Star Publishing Co

2. Dasgupta LR, Sundaraj T & Agarwal SC. (1974) Actinomycetes from myctomas and other cases around Pondichery. Indian J Med Res 62, 765-775.

3. De Hoog GS, Guarro J. (1995) Atlas of Clinical Fungi, pp 67, 69, 71, 76, 131, 132, 162, 179, 376. Centraalbureau voor Schmimelcultures, Baarn and Delft, The Netherlands

4. Gugnani HC, Ojukwu JO & Suseelan AV (1982) Mycetoma of the thumb caused by *Nocardia transvalensis*. Mycopathologia 80. 55-60

5. Gugnani HC, Suseelan AV, Anikwe RM & Ojukwu J. (1981) Actinomycetoma in Nigeria. J Trop Med Hyg 84, 259-263.

6. Indira PU & Sirsi M (1965) Studies on maduromycosis. Indian J Med Res 56, 1265-1277.

7. Joshi K.R., Sanghvi A., Vyas MCR & Sharma J.C. (1987) Etiology and diagnosis of mycetoma in Rajasthan, India. Indian J Med Res 85, 694-698.

8. Kandhari KC, Mohapatra LN, Sehgal VN & Gugnani HC. (1964) Black grain mycetoma of foot. Arch Derm 89, 867-770.

9. Koshi G, Padhye AA, Ajello, Chandler FW. *Acremonium recefei* as an agent of mycetoma in India. Amer J Trop Med Hyg (1979) 28, 692-696.

10. Koshi G, Victor N & Chacko J. (1972) Causal agents in mycetoma of the foot in Southern India. Sabouraudia, 10,14-18.

11. Kwon-Chung KJ, Bennett, J.E. (1992) Medical Mycology. Lea & Febiger, Philadelphia PP 560-593.

12. Land GA. (1996) Identification of aerobic actinomycetes in Clinical Microbiology Procedures Handbook (Ed. H.D. Isenberg), pp 4.1.1-4.1.9. American society for Microbiology, Washington, DC.

13. Mahgoub ES, Murray IG. (1973) Mycetoma William Heineman Medical Book, London

14. McGinnis MR. (1980) A Handbook of Medical Mycology, pp20, 166-169, 26-269, 507,508. Academic press, London

15. McNeil MM, Brown JM. (1994) The medically important aerobic actinomycetes: epidemiology and microbiology. Clin Microbiol Rev 7, 357-417.

16. Mishra SK, Gordon, RE & Barnett, DA. (1980) Identification of nocardiae and streptomycetes of medical importance. J Clin Microbiol 11, 728-736.

17. Pankajlaksmi VV, & Taralakshmi, V.V. (1984) Mycetomas in the tropics. Indian J Pathol. Microbiol 27, 223-228 .

18. Rippon JW. (1988) Medical Mycology, The Pathogenic Fungi and the Pathogenic Actinomycetes, pp. 80—118. W.B. Saunders Co..

19. Sandhu, DK, Mishra SK, Damodaran VN, Sandhu RS & Randhawa HS. (1975) Mycetoma of the knee due to *Nocardia caviae*. Sabouraudia 13,170-171.

20. Sanyal M, Thammaya A & Basu N. (1978) Actinomycetoma caused by the organisms of the *Nocardia asteroides* complex and closely related organisms. Mykosen 21, 109-121.

21. Thammaya A & Sanyal M. (1973) *Monosporium apiospermum* causing mycetoma pedis in India. Indian J Med Res 61, 1289-12291.

22. Thammaya A & Sanyal M. (1980) *Exophiala jeanselmei* causing mycetoma in India. Sabouraudia 18, 91-95.

23. Verghese A & Klokke AH. (1996) Histological daignosis of species of species of fungus causing mycetoma. Indian J Med Res 54, 524-530.

Mycetoma Plate: 1

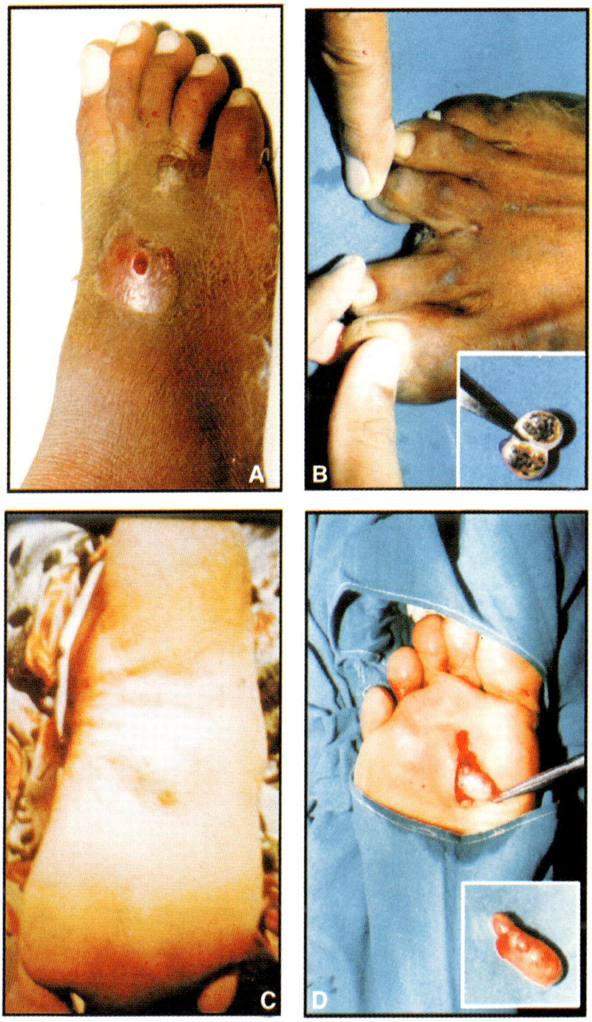

A. Mycetoma dorsum of foot showing swelling, sinuses and discharge of yellowish white granules

B. Mycetoma at interdigital site between toes showing swelling sinuses and discharge of black granules and cut section of cystic lesion showing black granules.

C. Mycetoma on planter surface of foot showing localised nodules with sinuses.

D. Localised cystic mycetoma without sinuses in subcutaneous tissue on planter site of foot and Removed cystic lesion showing nodules on the surface.

Mycetoma   Plate: 2

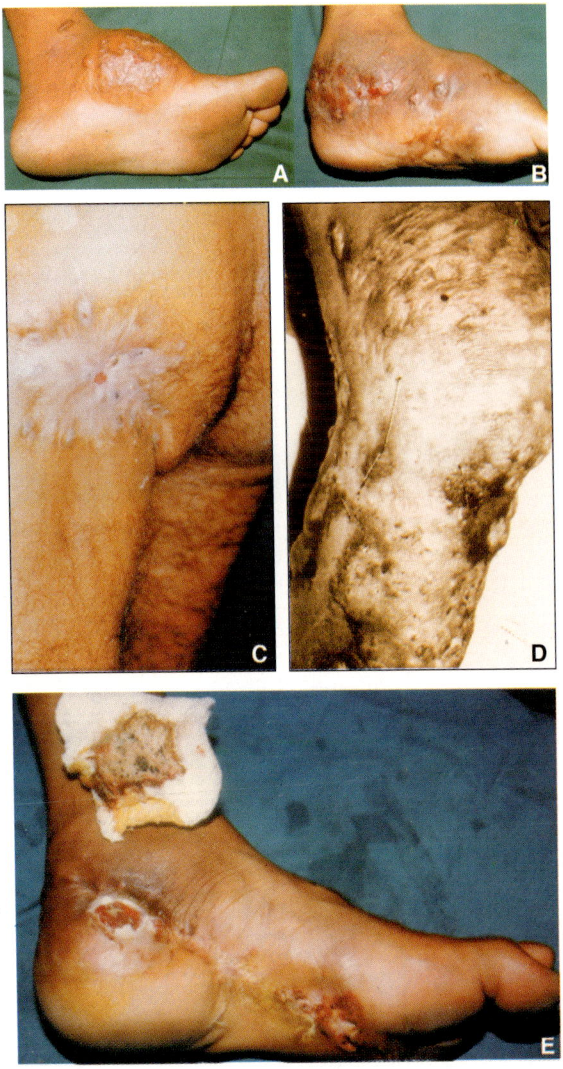

A. Mycetoma foot on dorsal and medial aspect with clinical cardinal signs.

B. Mycetoma foot with classical club shape foot having swelling and sinuses at all surfaces.

C. Mycetoma gluteal region.

D. Mycetoma knee involving surrounding area.

E. Mycetoma foot on planter and medial aspect showing recurrence over the previous operated site with discharged black granules on dressing.

Mycetoma Plate: 3

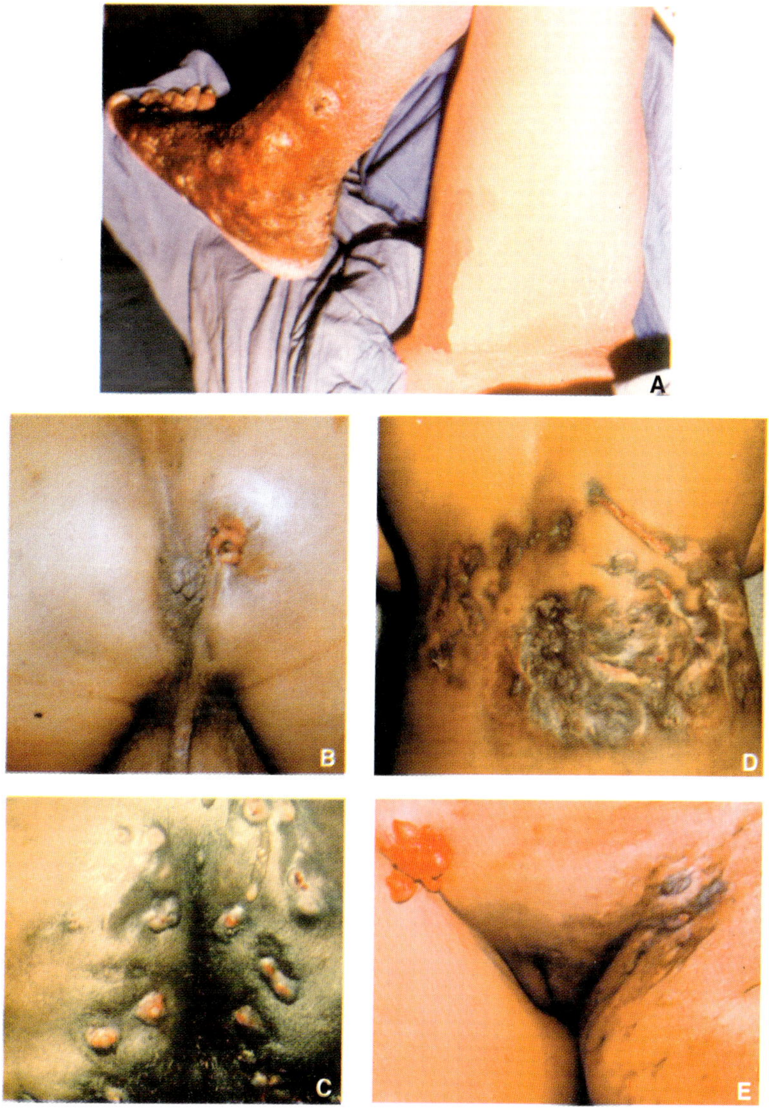

A. Mycetoma foot with sinuses and enlarged inguinal lymph node.

B. Mycetoma at perianal region.

C. Mycetoma perineum showing multiple sinuses.

D. Mycetoma back involving lumbar region.

E. Mycetoma upper part of thigh and inguinal region.

Mycetoma Plate: 4

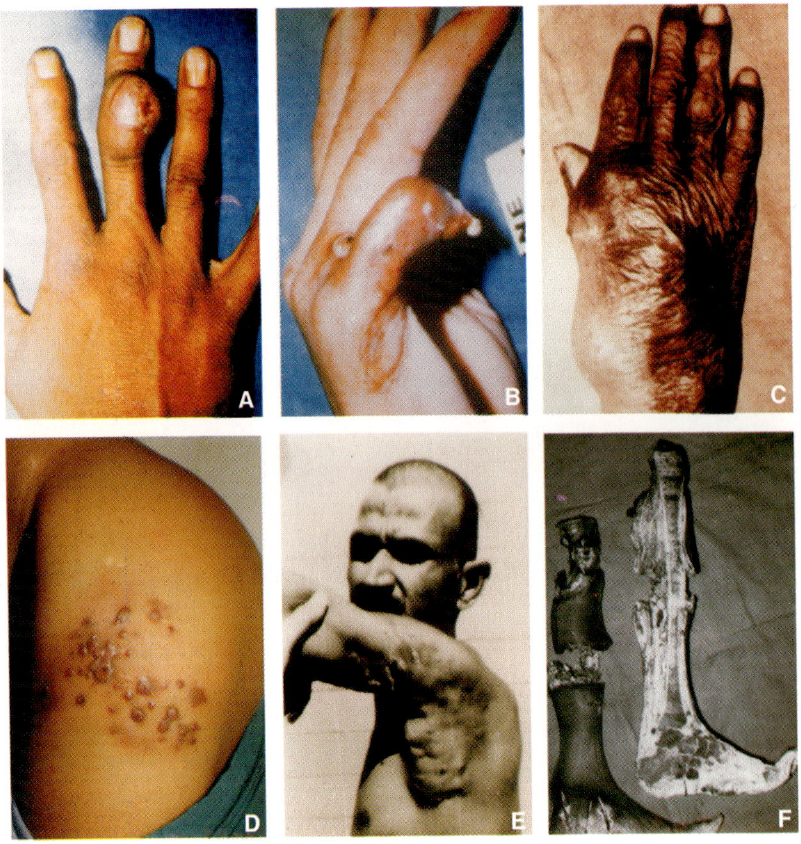

A. Mycetoma middle finger

B. Mycetoma little finger, interdigital space and adjacent palm area.

C. Mycetoma hand showing typical club shape swelling and sinuses.

D. Mycetoma shoulder region.

E. Mycetoma axilla and scapular region.

F. Dissected leg and foot of disarticulated limbs showing spread of mycetoma in muscles and bones.

Mycetoma Plate: 5

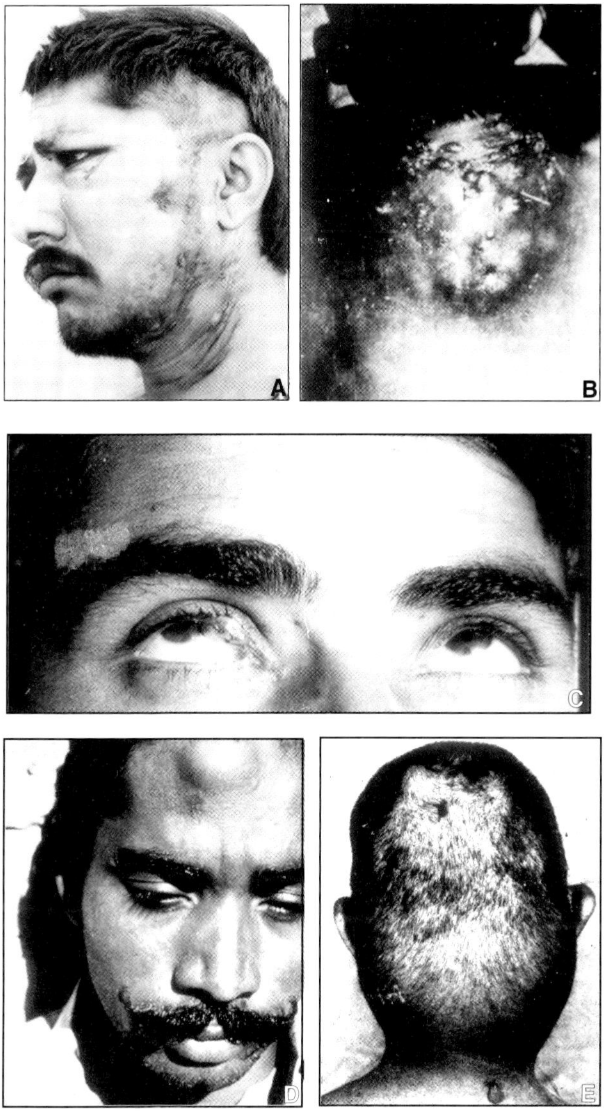

A. Mycetoma face and enlarged submandibular lymph nodes.

B. Mycetoma back of neck.

C. Mycetoma eye lid

D. Mycetoma fore head showing nodule without sinuses which showed granules when excised.

E. Mycetoma scalp involving its lower portion and posterior part of neck.

Mycetoma Plate: 6

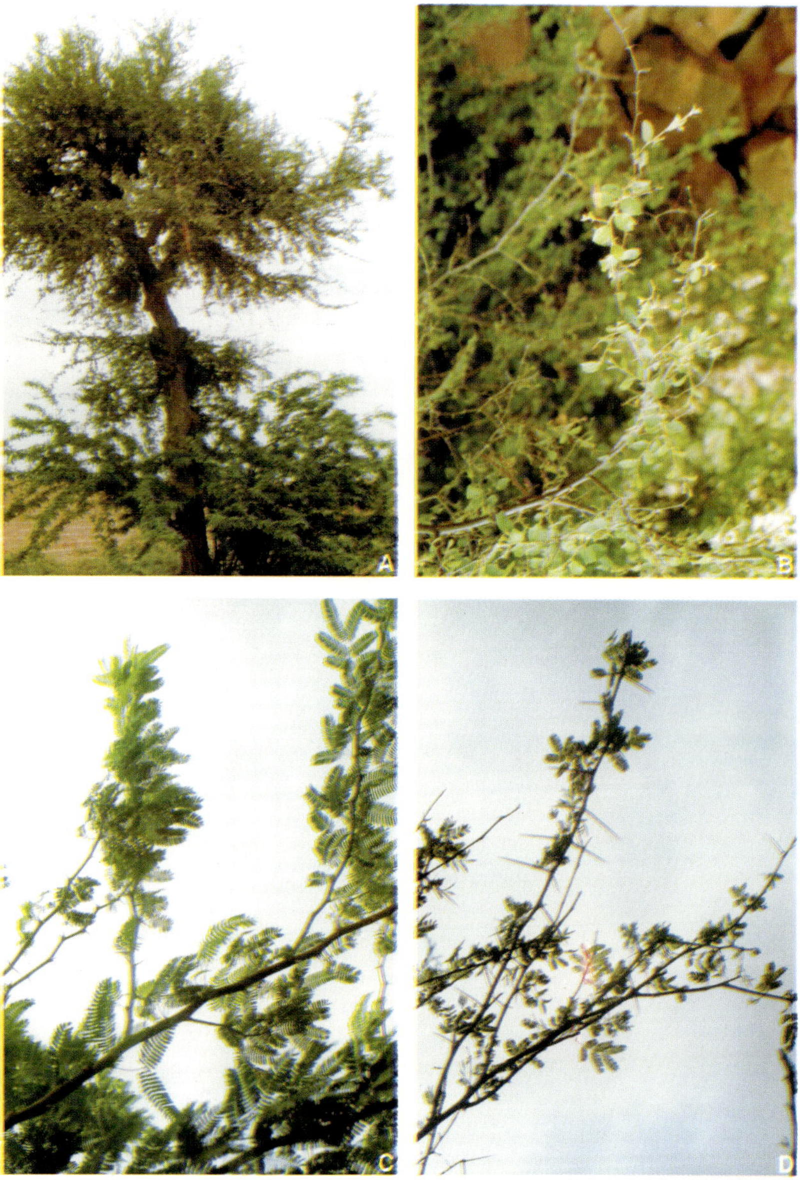

A. *Prosopis cineraria* (Khejdi)

B. *Ziziphus numularia* (Bair)

C. *Prosopis juliphora* (English Babul)

D. *Acacia nylotica* (Desi Babul)

Mycetoma Plate: 7

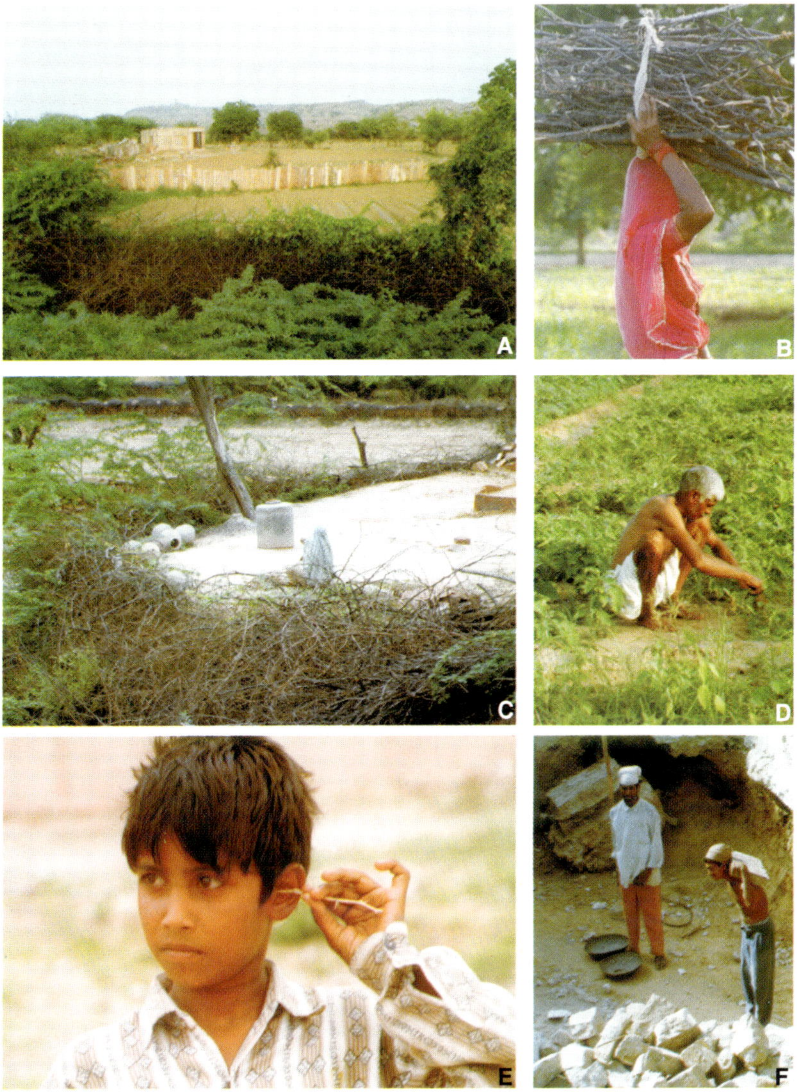

A. Field boundary of thorny twigs.

B. Lady carrying thorny twigs on head-scalp at risk of getting injury.

C. Lady sitting near boundary made of thorny twigs.

D. Field worker-working in squatting position-foot, hand and buttocks are at high risk of getting injury.

E. Child putting twig in ear to clean ear which is at risk of getting injury.

F. Labourer carrying stone on back - back and neck at risk of getting injury.

Mycetoma — Plate: 8

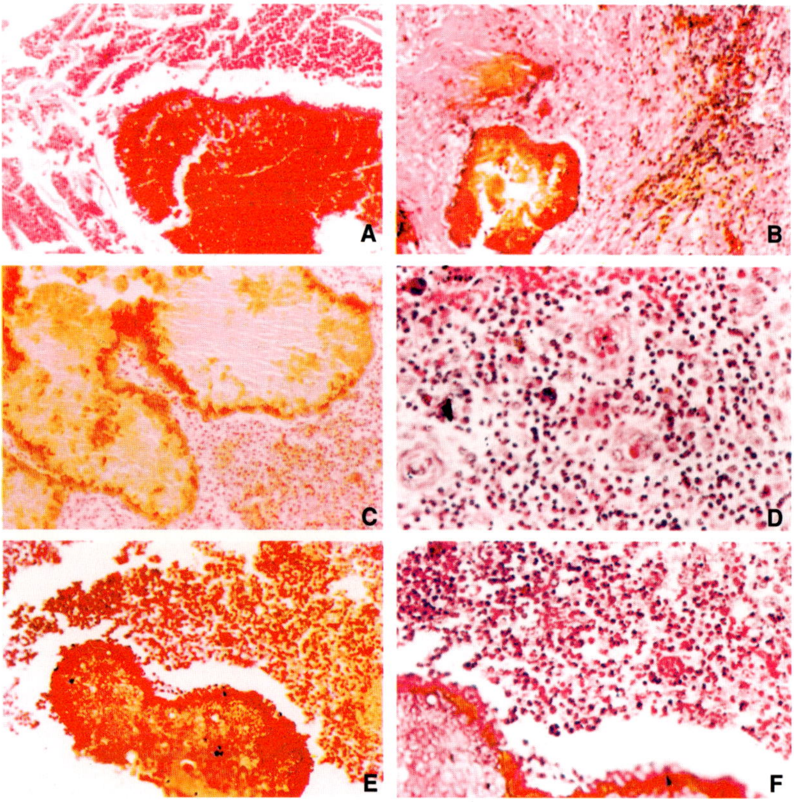

A. Madurella mycetomatis HE, 100X

B. Epithelioid cell reaction around granule of Madurella mycetomatis HE, 100X

C. Madurella grisea HE, 100X

D. Mixed inflammatory response with giant cell possibily containing fungal element in M.mycetomatis. HE, 450X

E. Exophiala jeanselmei, HE, 100X

F. Mixed inflammatory cell response around granule of Expohiala jeanselmei HE, 450X

Mycetoma Plate: 9

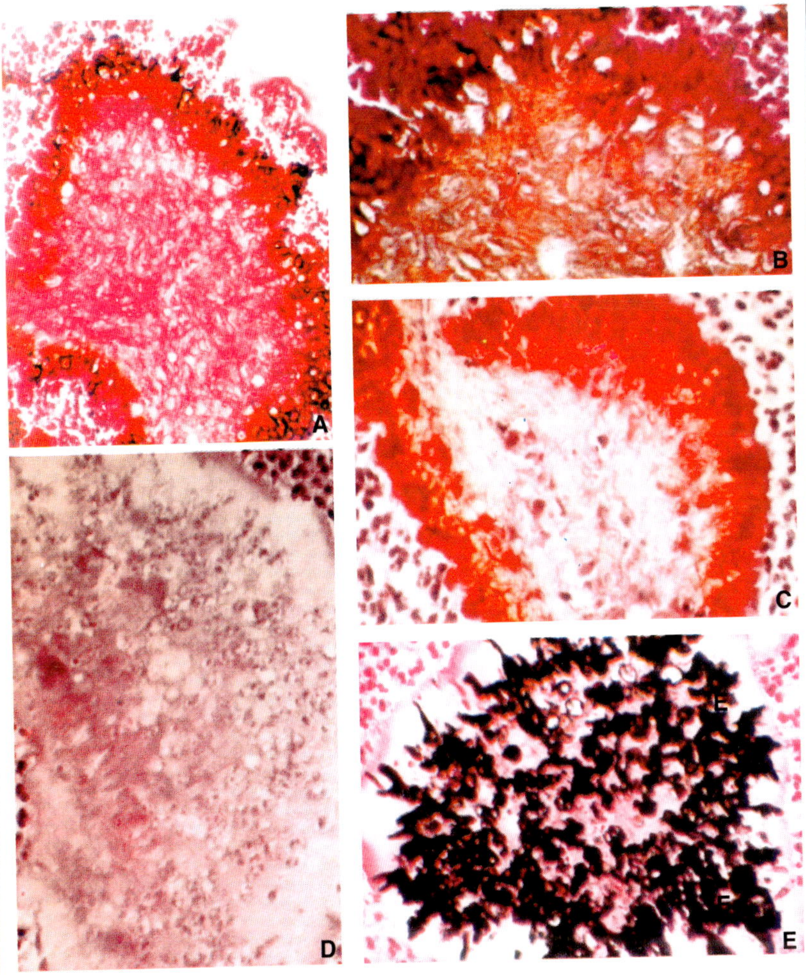

A. *Leptospheria senegalensis* granule showing dark periphery of dematiaceous mycelium with nonpigmented central part HE 50X

B. *Leptospheria senegalensis* showing higher magnification HE 100X

C. Pyrenochaeta romeroi- The outline of granules is curvilinear with darker periphery and lighter centre HE 100X

D. *Neotestudina rosatii*- The irregularly shaped granule composed of readily visible hyphae HE 100X

E. *Neotestuding rosatii*- GMS positive chlamydospores element within the granule and fer chlamydospores GMS HE 100X

Mycetoma Plate: 10

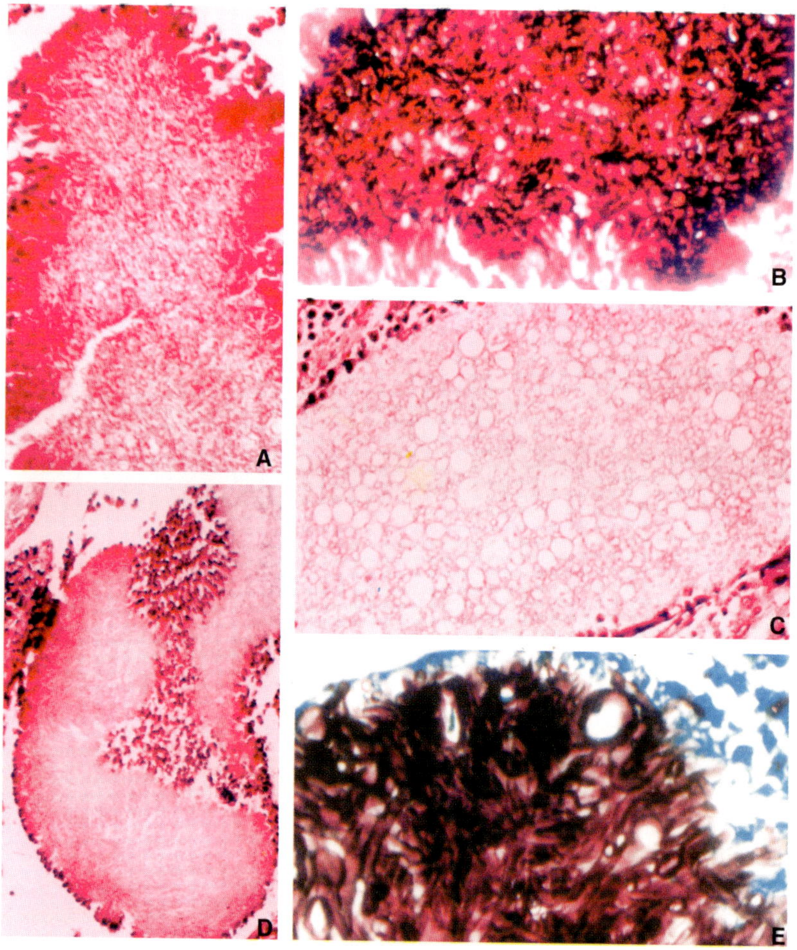

A. *Acremonium falciforme* showing network of mycelium and chlamydospores with prominent eosinophilic border H.E. 100X

B. *Acremonium falciforme* showing better visualisation of mycelium and chlamydospore in GMS-HE staining 100X

C. *Allescheria boydii*- The granule composed of mycelium and numerous large chlamydospores H.E. 100X

D. *Acremonium recifei*- The large granule hyaline mycelium, small chlamydospores with an eosinophilic border H.E. 50X

E. *Acremonium recifei*- The granule composed of mycelium and few chlamydospores GMS-HE 200X

Mycetoma Plate: 11

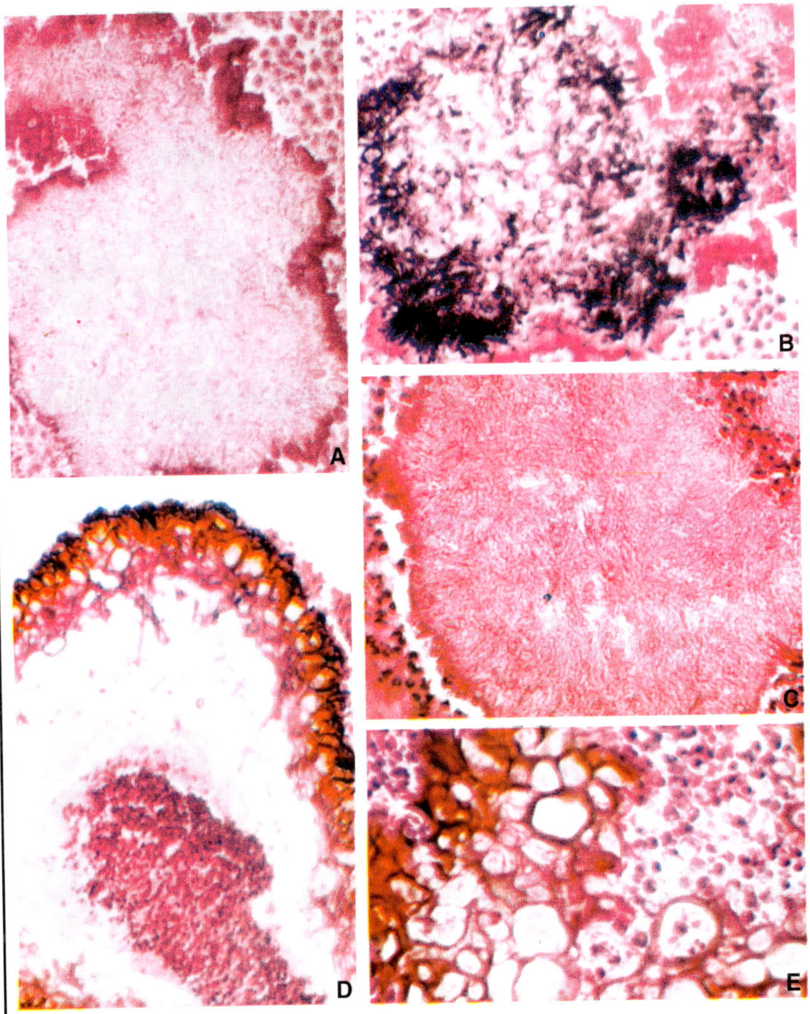

A. *Aspergillus nidulans*- The granule showing network of hyaline mycelium surrounded by eosinphilic border HE 100X

B. *Aspergillus nidulans*-The granule showing prominent esoinophilic border and network of hyphae GMS-HE 100X

C. *Fusarium monilifirme*- The granule has network of mycelium and a few chlamydospores with eosinophilic border HE 100X

D. *Curvularia geniculata*-The granule has peripheral dematiaceous mycelium and chlamydospores with central nonpigmented area. HE 50X

E. *Currularia geniculata*-Young granule embedded in microabscess showing fungal element in stage of development. HE 100X

Mycetoma

Plate: 12

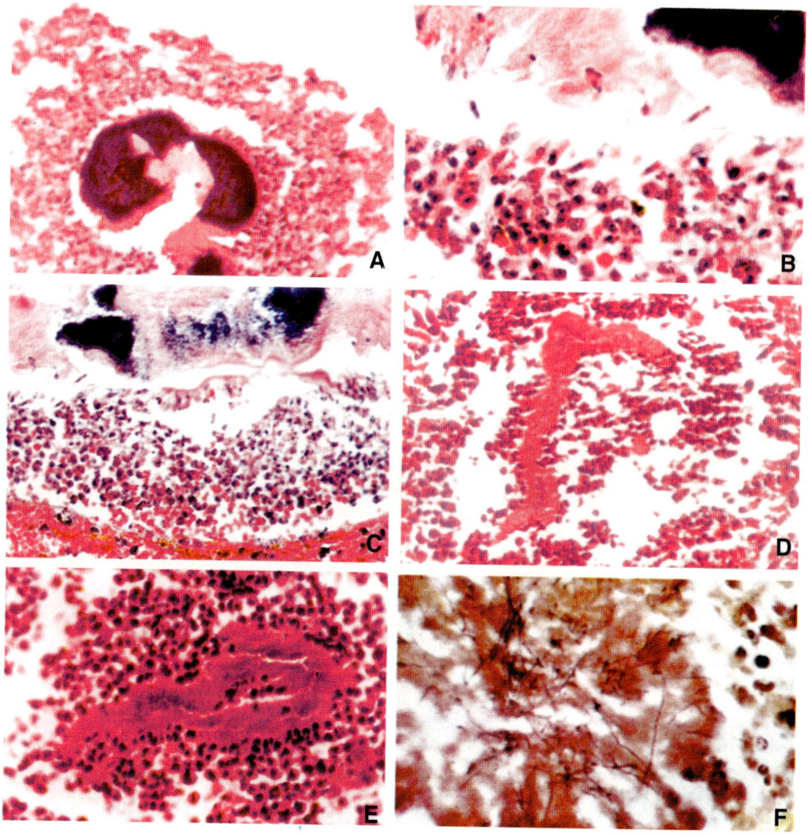

A. Acute inflammatory reaction around granule of Actinomadura madurae, HE, 100X

B. Acute inflammatory reaction around granules of Actinomadura madurae, HE, 450X

C. Actinomadura pellitieri HE, 100X

D. Nocardia Sp. HE, 100X

E. Acute inflammatory reaction around granule of Nocardia Sp. HE, 450X

F. Gram staining of granules of N. asteroids showing delicate branched mycelium with in the matrix of granule.

Mycetoma Plate: 13

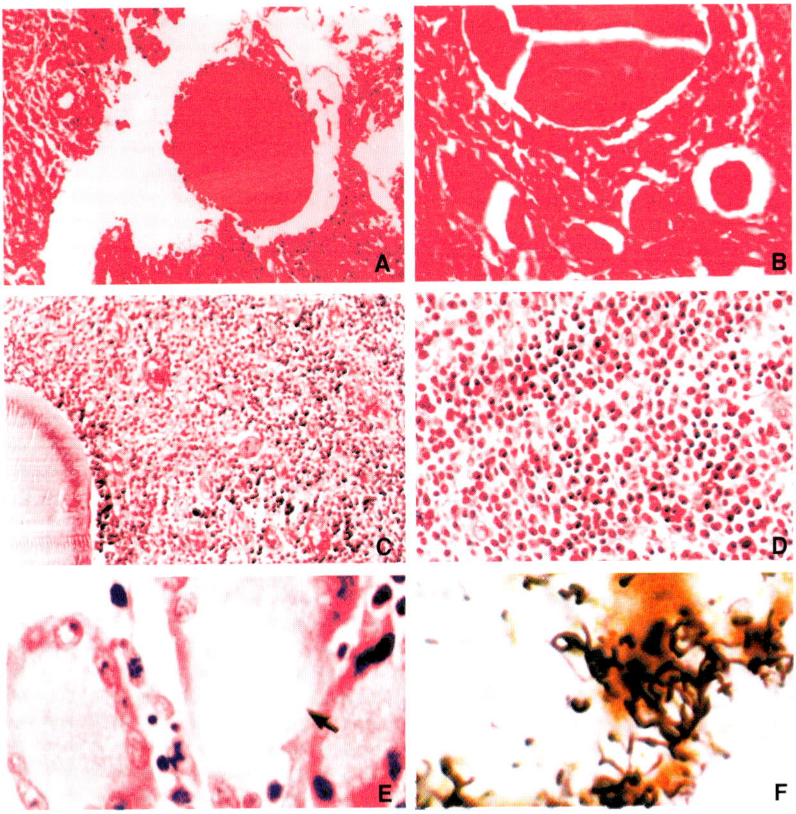

A. Streptomyces somaliensis, HE, 100X

B. Foreign body giant cell reaction around granule of Streptomyces somaliensis, HE, 450X

C. Vascular inflammatory mixed reaction with occasional foreign body giant cell around granules of Streptomyces somaliensis, HE, 100X

D. Predominantly plasma cell reaction away from granule of Streptomyces somaliensis. HE, 450X

E. Small granule of *S. somaliensis* engulfed by langhans' giant cell H.E. 200X

F. Delicate GMS positive filaments in granules of *S. somaliensis* GMS 500X

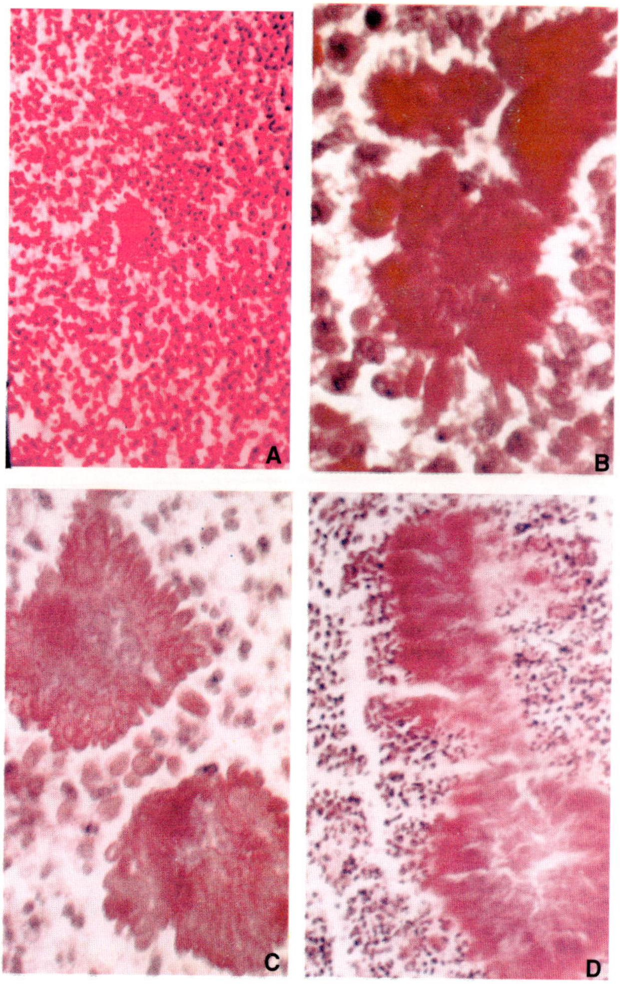

A. *Botryomycosis*- The granule is small with acute inflammatry reaction HE 100X

B. Botryomycosis caused by *Staphylococcus* sp. In higher magnification with purulent inflammatory reaction HE 200X

C. Botrymycosis caused by *Pseudomonas* sp.- The lighter basophillic granule is surrounded by prominent eosinophillic clubs at peripheral purulent infammatory reaction HE 200X

D. Botrymycosis caused by *Actinobacillus lignieresi*- The large irregular basophilic granule surrounded by esoinophilic border embedded in a abscess. HE 100X

Mycetoma Plate: 15

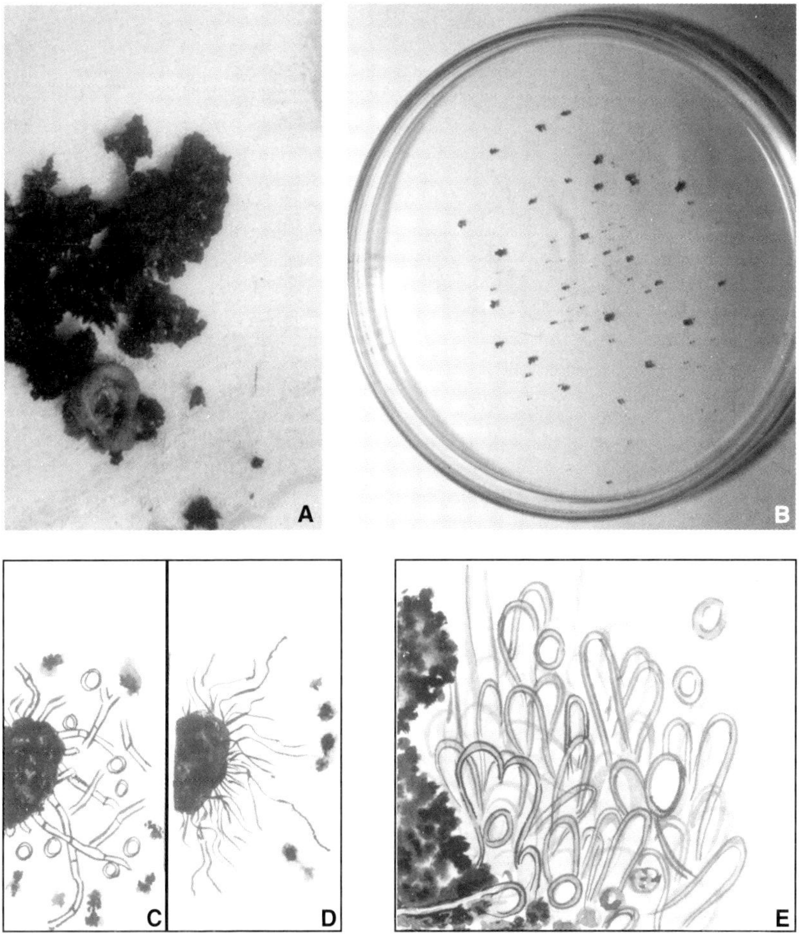

A. Black granules of Madurella mycetomatis from cystic lesion of mycetoma.

B. Scattered black granules of Madurella mycetomatis showing irregular size and shape.

C. KOH mount of crushed eumycetoma granules showing septate hyphae and chlamydospores.

D. KOH mount of crushed Actinomycotic mycetoma granules showing only thin mycelia.

E. KOH mount of crushed granules of Nocardia brasiliensis showing peripheral clubs of varying size.

Mycetoma Plate: 16

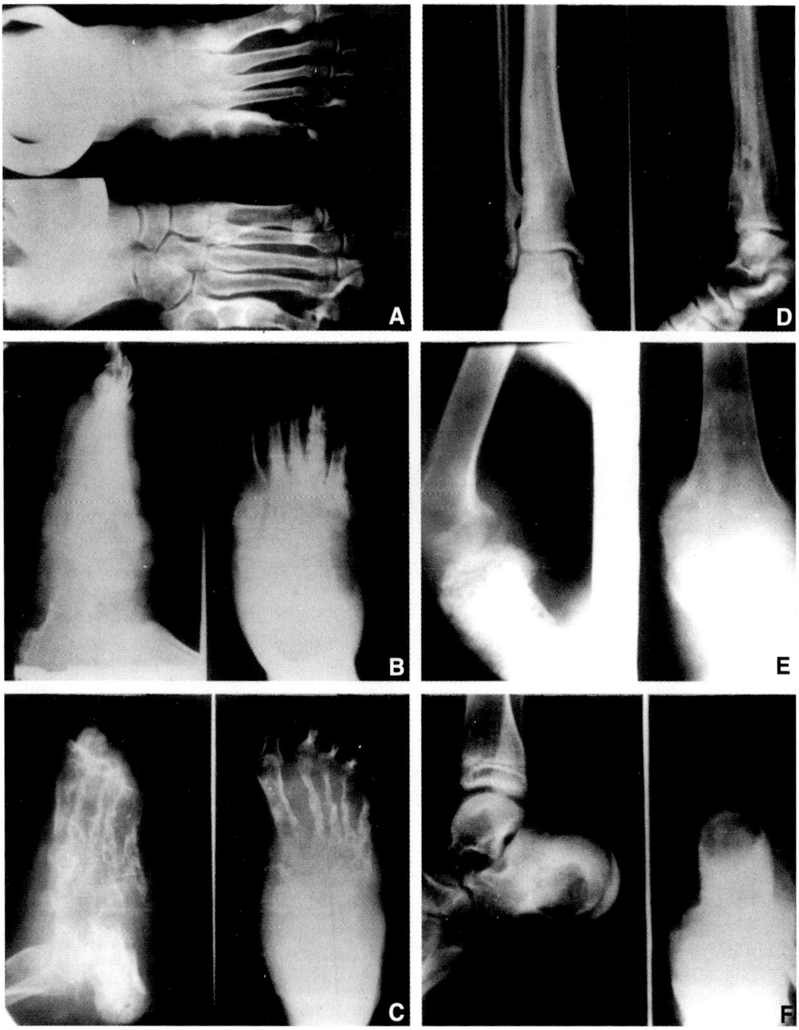

A. Eumycetoma foot showing ragged erosion of cortex from without.

B. Actinomycotic mycetoma foot showing periosteal reaction in the form of spicules projecting perpendicular to the line of cortex.

C. Advanced stage of eumycetoma foot showing excessive bone destruction and absorption of bones.

D. Eumycetoma leg recurred after treatment of mycetoma foot.

E. Actinomycotic mycetoma of upper end of tibia and knee joint.

F. Eumycetoma calcaneum.

Mycetoma Plate: 17

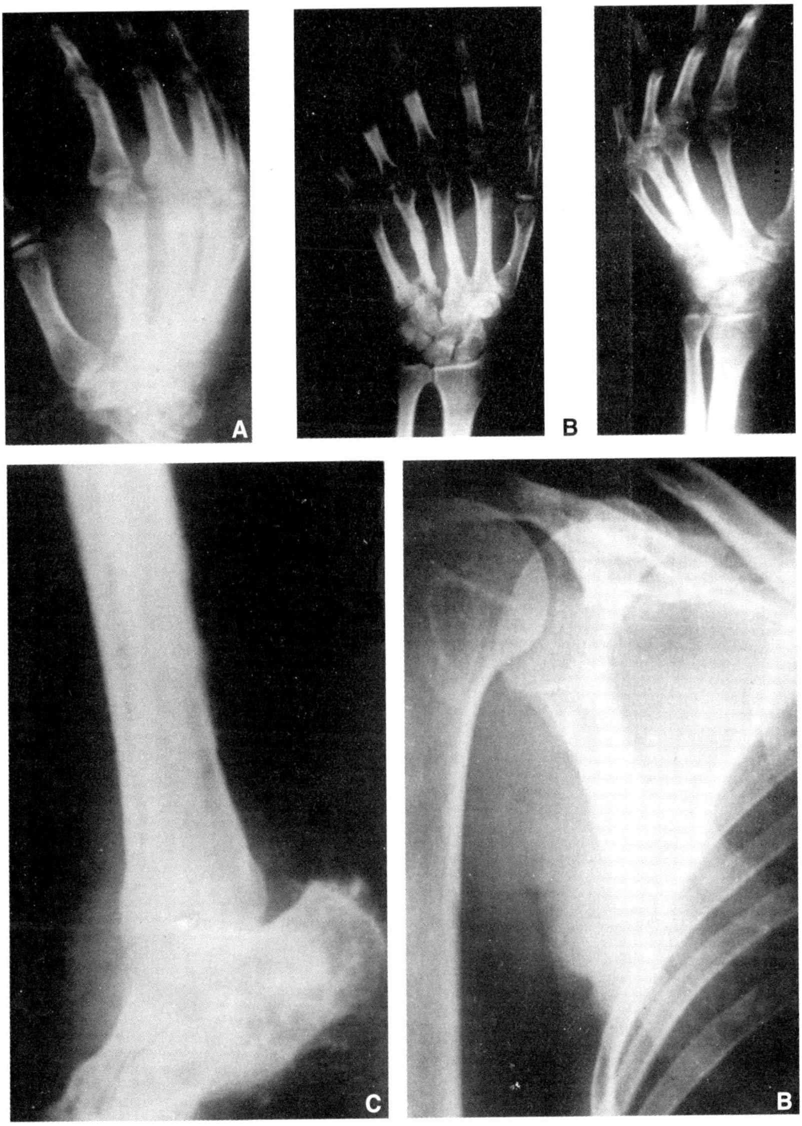

A. Actinomycotic mycetoma hand.

B. Eumycetoma hand showing thining of cortex and increased metacarpal space.

C. Actinomycotic mycetoma ankle joint and calcaneum.

D. Actinomycotic mycetoma involving scapular region.

Mycetoma Plate: 18

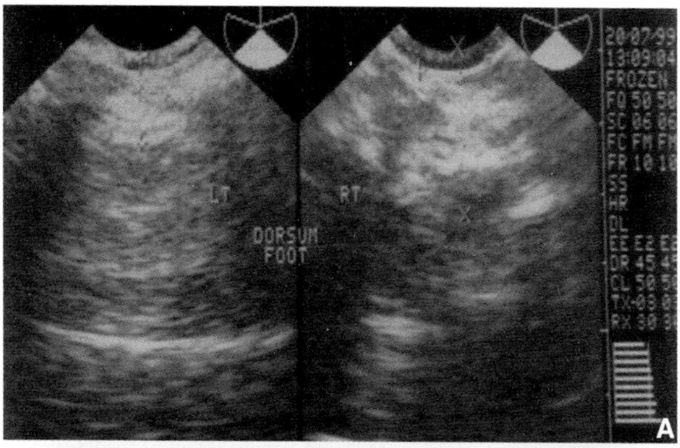

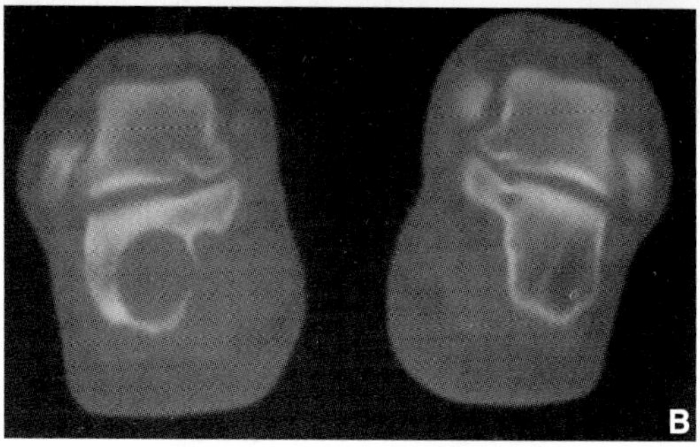

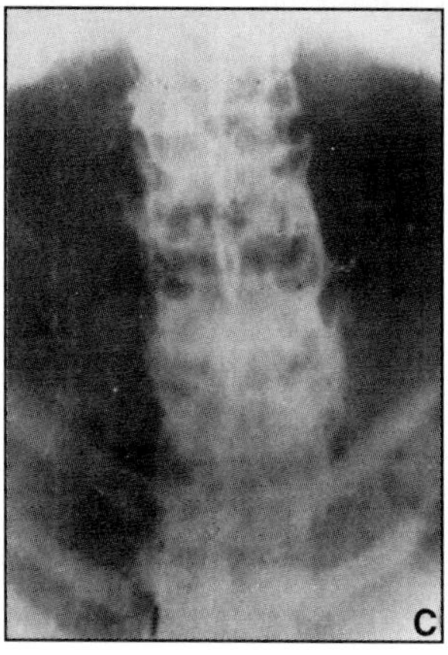

A. Sonography of dorsum of right foot showing hyper - reflective echoes with no acoustic enhancement.

B. C.T. Scan of operated foot showing "Weaver bird nest appearance".

C. Actinomycotic mycetoma of back involving vertebral column.

Mycetoma Plate: 19

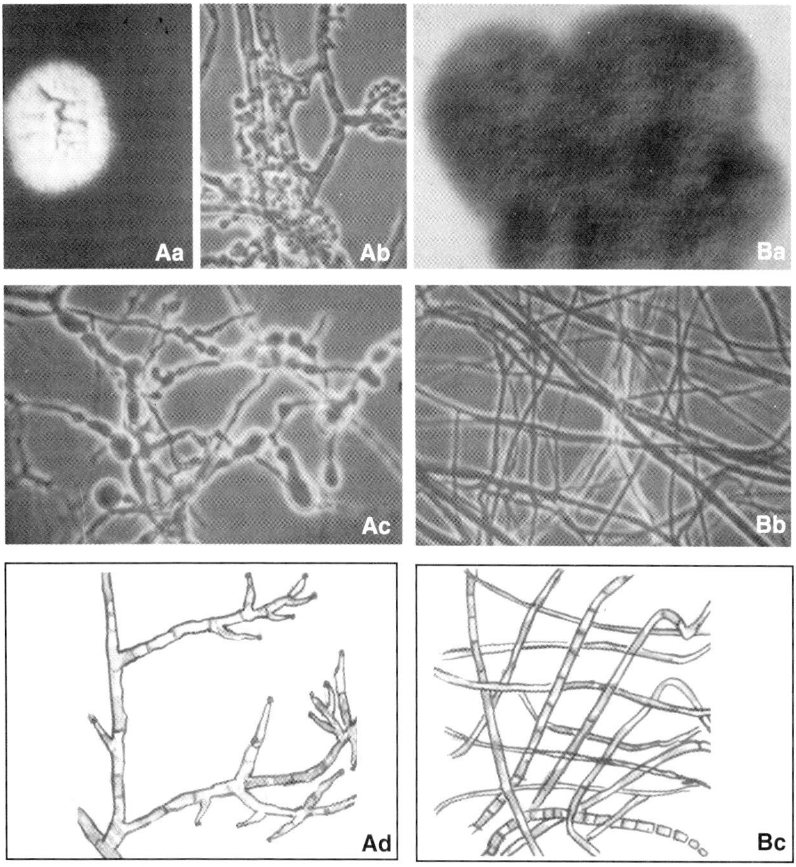

A. Madurella mycetomatis

a Colony

b Sporulation showing phialides and phialospores.

c Chlamydospores

d Line diagram showing phialides

B Madurella grisea

a Colony

b Non sporulating thin and thick hyphae.

c Line diagram showing nonsporulating thin and thick hyphae.

Mycetoma — Plate: 20

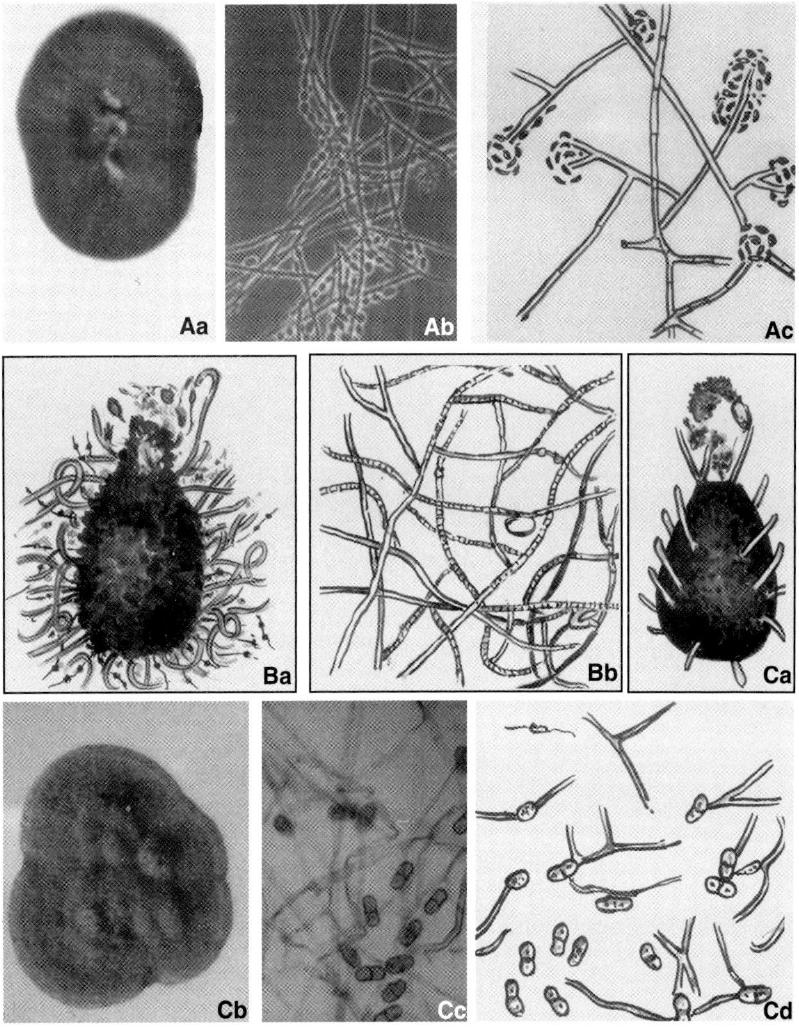

A. ***Exophiala jeanselmei:*** (a) Colony; (b) Moniliform hyphae; (c) Line diagram showing phialides and conidia

B. ***Leptosphaeria senegalensis:*** (a) Line diagram showing perithecium; (b) Line diagram showing septate hyphae.

C. ***Pyrenochaeta romeroi:*** (a) Line diagram of pycnida; (b)Colony; (c)Pycnospores; (d) Line diagram of pycnospores.

Mycetoma Plate: 21

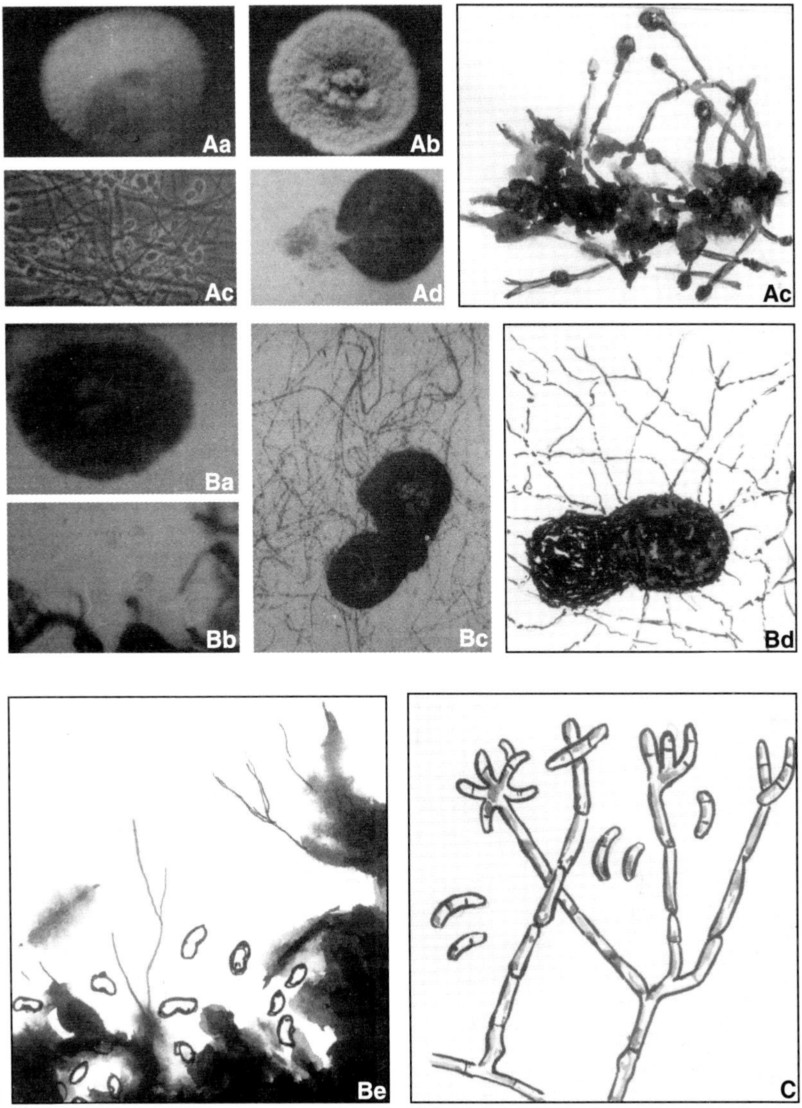

A. ***Pseudallescheria boydii*:** (a&b) Colonies; (c) Conidia and condiophores; (d) Ruptured ascocarp; (e) Line diagram of conidia and conidiophores.

B. ***Neotestudina rosatii*:** (a) Colony; (b) Ascospores from ruptured ascocarp (cleistothecia); (c) Ascocarp and hyphae; (d) Line diagram showing ascocarp and hyphae; (e) Line diagram showing ruptured ascocarp and ascospores.

C. **Acremonium falciforme** - Line diagram showing phialides and conidia.

Mycetoma Plate: 22

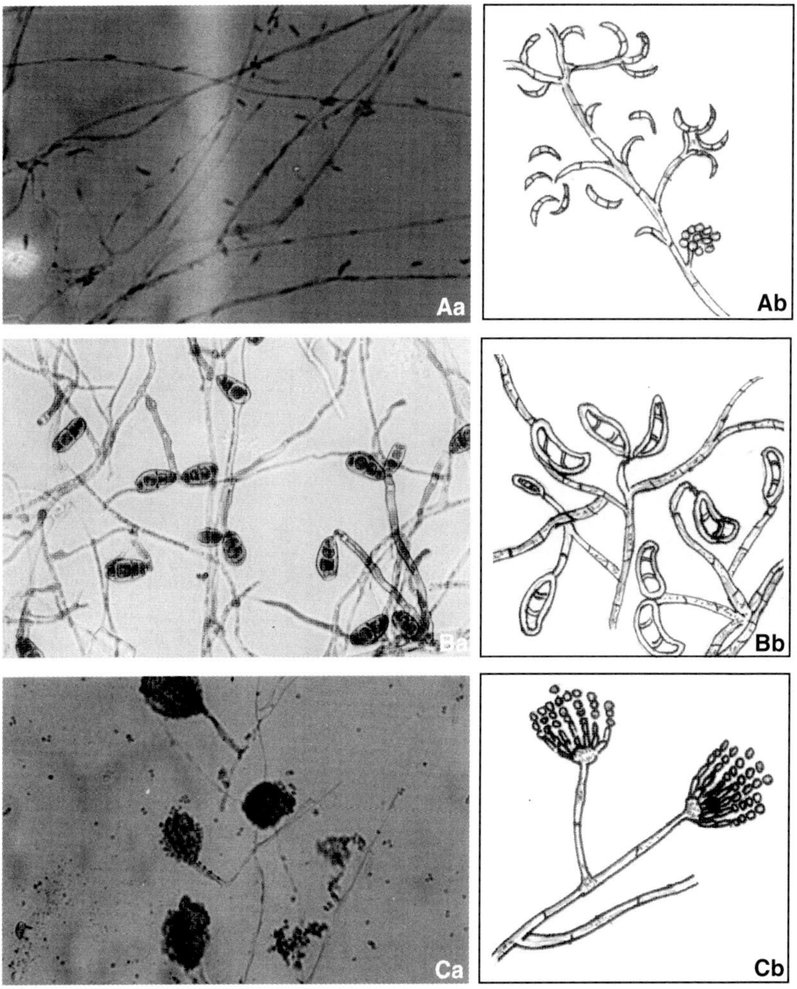

A. Fusarium species: (a) Fusarium species showing crescent shaped macroconidia; (b) Line diagram showing macroconidia and microconidia of Fusarium

B. Curvularia species: (a) Curvularia species showing septate brown hyphae and curved conidia; (b) Line diagram showing septate hyphae, conidiophores and curved conidia.

C. Aspergillus nidulans: (a) Aspergillus nidulans showing vesicle, phialides and conidia; (b) Line diagram of Aspergillus nidulans showing expanded conidiophore called vesicle, metulae, phialide and conida.

Mycetoma Plate: 23

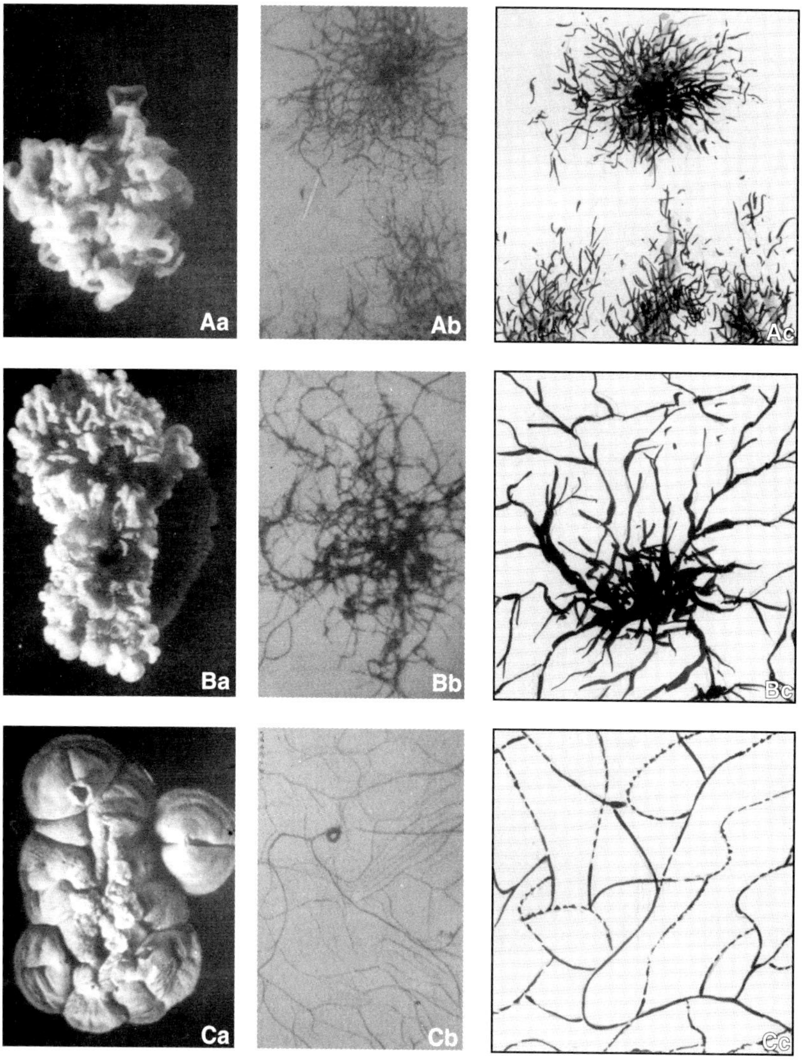

A. *Actinomadura madurae*: (a) Colony; (b) Thin mycelia; (c) Line diagram showing thin branched mycelia

B. *Actinomadura pellitieri*: (a) Colony; (b) Branched thin mycelia; (c) Line diagram showing thin branched mycelia

C. *Nocardia brasiliensis*: (a) Colony; (b) Thin branched; (c) Line diagram showing branched thin broken mycelia.

Mycetoma   Plate: 24

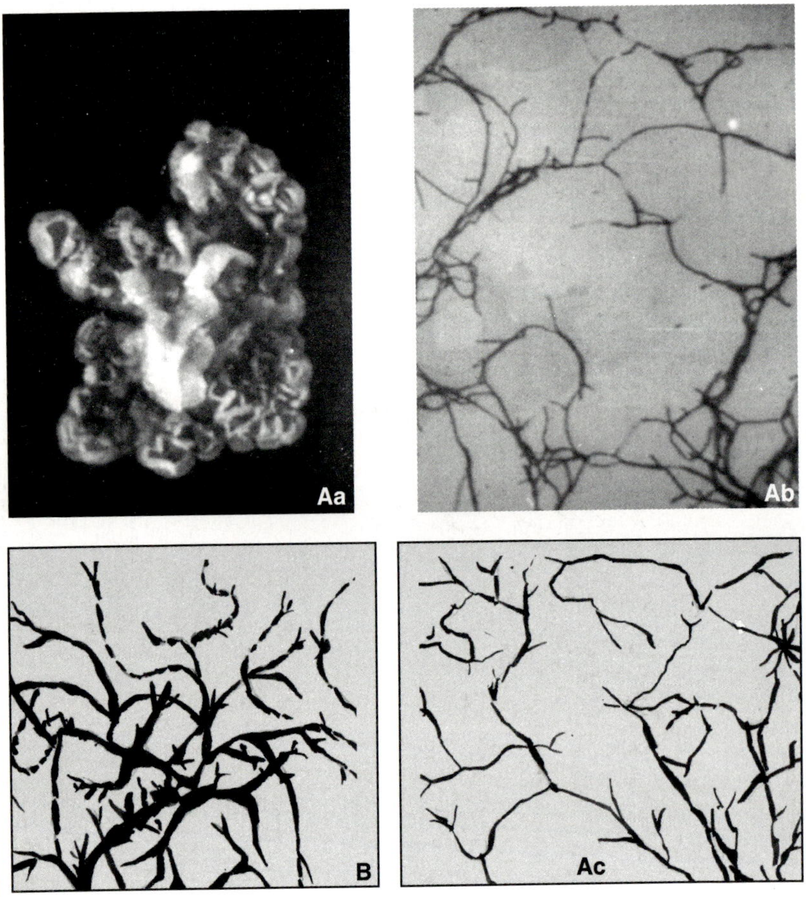

A. Streptomyces somaliensis

   a. Colony

   b. Mycelia

   c. Line diagram showing thin branched mycelia.

B. Nocardia caviae - Line diagram showing branched thin mycelia broken at ends.